LIVING LEAN
BY CHOOSING MORE

LIVING LEAN
BY CHOOSING MORE

Cheryl Jennings-Sauer

TAYLOR PUBLISHING COMPANY
Dallas, Texas

Designed by Bonnie Baumann
Illustrations by Robin H. Roberts

Published by Taylor Publishing Company
      1550 West Mockingbird Lane
      Dallas, Texas 75235

Library of Congress Cataloging-in-Publication Data

Jennings-Sauer, Cheryl.
   Living lean by choosing more.

   Includes index.
   1. Reducing diets.   2. Reducing exercises.
3. Health.   I. Title.
RM222.2.J47   1989   613.2   88-24823
ISBN 0-87833-604-4

Printed in the United States of America·

10 9 8 7 6 5 4 3 2 1

To my wonderful husband Robert,
who always seems to be there
when I need him most.

Acknowledgments

When it comes to big projects, we get by with a *lot* of help from our friends. Thanks to Mom and Wook, for your assistance at the drop of a hat; to Dee, Dad, and Evelyn, for your encouragement; and to Robin, for illustrating life into the text. More thank-yous are due Mary, Celeste, and Donna, for your hours of donated time.

I'm very grateful to Pat and Mike for getting the ball rolling, and to the wonderful supporting cast in order of appearance: Freddie, Alana, Melissa, and Alison. I also appreciate the time spent by Dr. Jack Wilmore of the University of Texas in reviewing the fitness section of the manuscript. Last, a very special thanks to Dudley Jahnke and the entire crew at Taylor Publishing for your extra effort and enthusiasm in anchoring a long, tough project.

Preface

. . . The only way is to eat less and exercise more.
—*The American Medical Association*

If you've heard such advice once, you've probably heard it a thousand times. Unfortunately, most of us have internalized only the first half of this maxim as our prescription for weight control. It's simply easier to eat less than to do more—no perspiration, no schedule alterations, no vicious dogs chasing us down the street. And since we feel a twinge or two of guilt about slighting the aerobic activity, we place double emphasis on cutting down in atonement.

Now consider this: the average adult's calorie consumption has declined over the past half century while average body weight has done just the opposite. Most women don't even eat the minimum number of recommended calories per day, yet they are still trying to fend off fat they don't want. This staggering blow is followed by a knockout punch: most of the same women—and a growing number of men—are on the verge of not getting enough of critical nutrients like vitamin B_6, iron, zinc, folacin, calcium, and magnesium, partly—if not primarily—due to their skimpy calorie consumption. Meanwhile, decreased physical activity is conspiring to maintain their calorie and nutrient intake at this close-to-inadequate level. "Obesity is a major malnutrition problem," states a nutrition textbook. Yet few overfat folks look in the mirror and murmur, "Boy, am I malnourished." And going on a diet (i.e., cutting calories still *further*) remains the most popular cure for unwanted fat.

To hear Living Lean students talk, however, you'd think all those diets were pretty dismal; "hungry," "deprived," "headache," "boring," and "temporary" are typical word associations. You can find a multitude of "diets" on any newsstand, and they sound great in theory. But most do not allow for individual differences or promote real changes in habits or lifestyle. They eventually self-destruct, torpedoing self-esteem at the same time. Here are just a few of the comments of some discouraged dieters:

> I did great on my diet all week long, but then our company picnic was Saturday and I had a big helping of pie. I knew I had blown the diet, so I kept on eating anything and everything all weekend. Now I'm really depressed. (Monica, a bookkeeper)

> The only time I become fixated on food and can't stop thinking about it is when I'm trying to follow a diet. That's crazy, isn't it? (Johnny, a sales manager)

> My husband weighs 220 pounds and they gave him a 1,000-calorie diet. The poor man nearly starved to death. (Lorraine, a loving spouse)

Although medically supervised low-calorie dieting and fasting are appropriate for extremely overfat patients, moderately overfat people need a fat-loss technique that is safe and workable with little or no professional monitoring. After all, every dieter is destined to be on his or her own sooner or later.

Living Lean was specifically designed to satisfy both of these criteria. Over the past eight years this program has expanded to include the five- to eight-week Living Lean Project™, Living Lean and Fit™, Lunch-Hour Lean™, and Living Lean workshops and seminars, in settings ranging from fitness facilities and small discovery groups to corporate wellness and hospital health promotion programs. Participants include college students, homemakers, career men and women, and recent retirees, with ages ranging from 17 to 72. Because of its health-building philosophy, Living Lean attracts athletes who take fitness seriously and people who haven't taken a recreational walk in years; formerly overfat folks who are now active and formerly active folks who are now overfat; people who can't find time to eat and those who eat all the time; natural-food lovers and junk-food junkies; adults with serious health problems and teenagers just recovering from bulimia; compulsive eaters who consume without thinking and conscientious dieters who have "tried everything." Within this diverse audience are many who are already lean and healthy—people who simply want a lean-maintenance program to ensure that vitality for the future.

To make their task a little easier, Living Lean students have repeatedly asked for a workbook to accompany the program as well as a do-it-yourself manual for interested friends and relatives. The book you are holding is the answer to their requests. At the same time, all these folks are savvy enough to know it's a challenge to live lean in the midst of plenty—there is no quick fix.

The good news is that winds of positive change are stirring. According to a Gallup survey, six of every ten people are now doing some sort of regular exercise; that's a "healthy" majority. If you don't fall in with the popular ranks soon, you're liable to get left behind. And there are other shifts. Fast-food eateries still push greasy burgers, but you can often find smaller portions, leaner meats, and fresh salad bars. It's no longer a contest to see how much you can drink before you pass out, either; instead it's how many miles you can run in 30 minutes flat.

The trend is so upbeat you might even see your aspirations change—from "ten pounds thinner" to "looking better, feeling great." Another bonus: many new habits will be self-perpetuating, thus easy to stick with. For instance, you may find nutritious food to be quite delicious, not distasteful, and aerobic activity to be pleasantly addictive rather than a boring chore.

Nor is it necessary to jog six miles a day or live on yogurt and wheat germ to notice improvements in your health. Instead, Living Lean encourages small successes, starting right where you are now. You can even go part-time on this project—Living Lean is equipped to handle an occasional splurge—so long as you remain wholehearted in your commitment. That's what Living Lean boils down to: a commitment to good health. Reading a book, joining a fitness club, even checking in at an expensive health spa won't do the trick unless some serious mental calisthenics precede the physical.

When it comes to their lifestyles, discriminating adults demand the freedom to make choices as well as the opportunity to make a few mistakes. To avert truly unnecessary blunders, the techniques that have worked best for the most people are outlined for you here in an eight-week, step-by-step action and eating plan. Living Lean recognizes that no two people are alike, so you will be encouraged to tailor suggested strategies to fit your own needs. There are ideas and exercises for people who appreciate detailed information, plus shortcuts for the "spare me the details, get to the point" types. Even those who are constitutionally opposed to following menu plans can still build health and burn fat by using the many qualitative changes set forth in this book.

The basic program philosophy is condensed into Living Lean's easy-to-remember Success Formula, Q^2FiT—which stands for Quality Control, Quantity Control, Fitness, Initiative, and Timing. You will be encouraged to eat high-fiber, nutrient-dense foods that are low in fat—not only to shrink body fat but to build health (Quality Control). If you move more, you can lose fat even without drastic calorie restriction; you'll learn how to determine the appropriate calorie intake for you based on your new activity level and body size (Quantity Control).

Overall fitness is the program's cornerstone, raising your fat-burning metabolism while preserving lean muscle (Fitness). Living Lean will also get you going and keep you going with attitude-adjusting and self-image-boosting techniques that really work (Initiative). And last, you'll plan an eating and activity schedule to enhance optimum fat loss (Timing).

Any one of these components could prove to be your Missing Link. When you discover it, you may find that the rest of the Success Formula falls into place with little additional effort. Your Missing Link could just as easily be something that interferes with the formula, breaking the functional chain. The "Spoilers"—sugar, salt, caffeine, and alcohol—can easily gum up the gears of your Living Lean machinery. Living Lean requires only that you identify major problem areas and work on those first. In the process, you may stumble across your personal Missing Link, saving yourself lots of misdirected effort.

As you discover what works, you'll also realize what doesn't. Forget the daily ritual of stepping on the scale as well as the restrictive calorie counting from your previous "deprivation diets." Like dinosaurs, such schemes are doomed to extinction. In contrast, you can rely on Living Lean as a perpetual partner, passing the torch to you at that point when you can trust your own body signals (and your newfound common sense) in deciding what, when, and how much to eat, with the ultimate goal of living independently healthy and "diet"-free.

When compared with typical "diets," Living Lean sounds like a genuine alternative. But is it the right alternative for you? If you are hunting for reliable advice on becoming lean and healthy, you will find it here. If you already know what to do and just aren't doing it, Living Lean may help you cross the bridge from inertia to initiative. If you are discouraged by past "diet" failures, Living Lean can restore your confidence (you didn't fail; the "diet" failed *you*).

If you are ready to assume responsibility for your health, then Living Lean is the right choice. More good food, more productive activity, and more exhilarating energy and enthusiasm are just a few of the rewards you can look forward to. And if you've been "dieting" more these days and disliking it more than ever, please read on. Living Lean has some good news for you!

> **A reminder:** You are unique, so check with your physician and professional nutritionist before beginning this program. The information presented here is intended as a general supplement to, not a specific substitute for, their advice and recommendations.

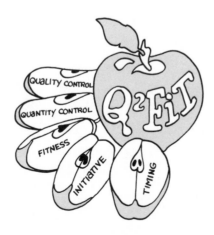

CONTENTS

Preface   vii

Introduction   xiii

WEEK ONE   1

It's About Time   1
Positively Speaking (and Thinking and Doing)   4
Medical Exam and Personal Health Record   6
Body Fat: Friend and Foe   7
Progress Evaluation   12
Get a Line on Labels   12
Eating Diary   16
Practice Diary One   16

WEEK TWO   20

What's the Verdict? Eating Diary Analysis   20
The Fiber Connection: Filling, Not Fattening   24
Tame Your Appetite   33
The Caffeine Scene   37
Practice Diary Two   39

WEEK THREE   42

Earn an "F" for Fabulous Fitness   42
Aerobic Engineering: Move It to Lose It   45
Living Fitness   53
Salt: Shake It Easy   59
Practice Diary Three   63

WEEK FOUR   66

Quality Control Assurance   66
Living Lean with *Less* Protein   80
Practice Diary Four   83

WEEK FIVE   86

Meet Your Metabolism   86
Fitness: Beyond Good Intentions   96
Sticks and Stones and Sturdy Bones   104
Practice Diary Five   107

WEEK SIX   110

Quantity Control Assurance   110
The Training Table: Practice Eating to Make Perfect   113
Practice Diary Six   141

WEEK SEVEN   144

Stress: Fix It before You Break   144
Speed Eating Is Not a Sport   151
Stalking Simple Sugars   153
Practice Diary Seven   159

WEEK EIGHT   162

Whatever Works—For *You*   162
Practice Diary Eight   165

Appendix A.   Body Fat Indicator   **169**
Appendix B.   Fitness Walking Test   **170**
Appendix C.   Resources   **174**
Index   **175**

Introduction

How to Make This Book Work for You

Unless someone has volunteered to do it for you, you are probably ready to become actively involved in your personal health and fitness project. In addition to the information and inspiration packed into *Living Lean by Choosing More*, there are also a lot of almost-blank pages—activity logs, weekly practice diaries, self-discovery exercises, and evaluative questionnaires. These pages will be the most significant portion of the book (they're noted with an asterisk [*] in the Table of Contents for each chapter), but only *after* they are completed by you.

Do you have a pencil with eraser in hand right now? It's a good idea to grab one whenever you pick up this book. You might believe you know what you think (and how you eat)—that is, until your thoughts climb out of your brain, slide down your pencil, and land on the paper. (The Eating Diary you will keep offers good examples of how your memory plays tricks on you.) Reading your impressions in vivid black and white will also help you deal with them critically and objectively.

Take your time with these exercises; unlike single-concept books that can be digested at one sitting, there is a lot of food for thought "sandwiched" in these chapters. If some idea really jumps out at you, put the book down for a while and let your subconscious focus on it—it could be especially important. Even better than an eight-week project is an eight-*month* project. Those months will go by anyway, so why not put them to good use? This is your venture; you decide whether you are worth the effort.

Feel free to use whatever strategies work best, but do give all the suggested practices at least one shot; working through the activities is more beneficial than skimming the book for basic information. In fact, several of the simple-sounding exercises, like the Pantry Inventory, have been rated as extremely valuable by Living Lean students.

Consider all the activities as experiments—some will work out, some won't. If you sense a lot of resistance when you are faced with a new idea, ask yourself, "Why am I rejecting this?" before totally passing it by. Rest assured all suggested practices are for one week only, to be extended solely at your option.

Be aware of your feelings as well as your thoughts during the coming weeks and jot them down if possible. Be honest; there's no need for anyone to see this book besides you, and you certainly wouldn't want to kid yourself. Some students set aside a quiet time for thinking about their Living Lean goals: on the bus to work, in the tub, or late at night. When you are relaxed, your subconscious will be more likely to pick up any positive messages or visual images you send it.

If you are a "professional dieter," you may have to deprogram your guilt feelings and food phobias that have been reinforced by years of thinking in terms of "forbidden" versus "recommended" food. Living Lean is a whole new ball game; you deserve to eat and to enjoy the dining experience. Food is not the enemy, it is your key to survival. You can't be healthy—or lean—without it.

What can you expect once you adopt the Living Lean lifestyle? *Unexpected* benefits. The combination of good nutrition, physical activity, and fresh air delivers what the fat-jiggling machines can't: a sly smile, extra vigor in your step, and a rosy blush on your cheeks. Like a rejuvenating weekend at a health resort, Living Lean helps you bring about a visible change; liberated from puffy eyes and swollen jowls, you can put your "best face" forward with newfound confidence. After only a week or two, don't be surprised if your friends exclaim, "Oh, you've lost weight!"—*before* any significant body fat (or weight) adjustments have taken place.

After this initial esteem-booster comes the nitty-gritty—body reshaping. It takes time (you knew that was coming!) to eliminate and redistribute surplus fat from years of inactivity. In the old days the bathroom scale was your only clue to success or failure in this department, but you need new criteria now. Instead of setting a target weight for yourself, create some action-oriented goals that refocus your attention away from the scale. For instance, you might decide to walk 45 minutes six times a week or to drink only one beer instead of two. Positive practice makes perfect, so record your action goals on the weekly Practice Diary at the end of each chapter and make an attempt to follow through. Decisions to try new routines are entirely at your discretion, and with the Practice Diary you get a check mark just for trying!

Your ultimate goal is to burn body fat without slowing your metabolism, jeopardizing your nutritional status, or burning out on the project. The following sequence of changes will lead you in the right direction.

- **Week One:** Your immediate task is to build a firm metabolic foundation. While you are getting psyched up to begin your lifetime of Living Lean, you should also get started on your fitness program.
- **Week Two:** By snacking more often and choosing more foods with fiber, you can add Quality Control as well as Quantity Control to your everyday eating—*without* counting calories. In conjunction with your fitness effort the two Q's will fire up the fat-burning process.
- **Week Three:** This week you get more detailed instruction for setting up a personalized fitness plan. Even if you are not aware of it, the changes you initiated during the previous two weeks are already beginning to regulate your appetite. Physical activity is truly the heart of the Living Lean program.
- **Weeks Four and Five:** You should begin to notice a reduction in body fat (and inches) by the fourth or fifth week even if your body weight is not yet changing. Chapter 5 shares some of the secrets for promoting fat-burning and lean-building metabolism; at the same time, eating, activity, and lifestyle changes are becoming more routine as health-defeating habits slowly fall away.
- **Weeks Six through Eight:** By this time, fat loss should register on your scale as well as your tape measure. Since physical results are likely to reflect physical effort, you may want to extend your aerobic excursions by 15 to 30 minutes. If you feel hungry much of the time, you may even need to *increase* your calories a bit to parallel the positive changes in your body composition and metabolism.
- **Beyond Eight Weeks:** If you continue to practice Quality Control in eating and maintain or step up your physical activity, your appetite will become a reliable indicator of how much you need to eat. From that point it's only a matter of time before Living Lean becomes second nature. Anyone can "lose" weight. But if you do it the Living Lean way, it's far less likely to "find" you again.

Does it really work? Living Lean principles and strategies are based not only on scientific research but also on what *has* worked for most participants. The following letter expresses the enthusiasm of one Living Lean "alumnus":

Dear Cheryl:

Your Living Lean program is certainly one of a kind. I have tried to lose weight for years, but never seemed to find anything that really made sense or worked long-term.

I am now happy to report that by living lean I have lost inches. My belt is five inches shorter than before and my cholesterol count continues to fall. One of the things that helped me to be open to trying to "live lean" was your method of presenting advice and information. You were not accusing or judgmental. When participants shared their successes or failures, you fed them honest facts and encouragement. Thanks for a good program that will be a permanent way of life for me.

Sincerely,
Kennith Langham

There are no gimmicks here, no pounds-lost-or-money-back guarantees. But if your lifetime goal is getting lean and living healthy, then choose the Success Formula that really works—you can *count* on Living Lean!

Sections of the book are marked with logos to help you use each part effectively. The following list explains these symbols:

Written Exercises

Practice

Recipes

Aerobictips

Label Lingo

The Progression toward Health and Fitness

You need plenty of effort, time, and patience to make the transition from overfat to lean and fit. Which of the following best describes your current status? Indicate with a check mark (✔).

☐ **Dissatisfaction and Rationalization**—leading gradually to the realization that being lean and healthy *may* be more rewarding than the aftereffects of eating whatever you want, whenever you want it, and being physically inactive. "It doesn't matter . . . "; "I'll just eat one or two . . . "; "I'm too tired . . . "

☐ **The Turning Point**—could be anything, such as a glance through an old photo album; chest pains while walking up the stairs; a return to being single after years of marriage; a thoughtless remark by some acquaintance.

☐ **Change and Practice**—given time, sufficient practice, and energy generated by the Turning Point, the changes evolve into a new status quo; old habits are seen more and more as negative, unhealthy, and unrewarding.

☐ **New Self-Image**—preceded by positive feelings and statements about yourself and distinct pleasure at what your body *is* and *can* do (in place of dwelling on what it *isn't* and *can't* do); the mental picture begins to reflect the true mirror image.

☐ **Adjusting**—includes splurging on food, but this time taking it in stride; accumulating some extra fat during a stressful time, then returning to a healthy routine; or weathering failures in a job or romance as a lean, healthy person, because a new and improved body doesn't guarantee a trouble-free existence.

WEEK ONE

It's About Time
  *Are You Game for Change?
  *Participation Agreement
  Treasure Mapping for Success

Positively Speaking (and Thinking and Doing)
  *Are You a Positive Person?

Medical Exam and Personal Health Record
  *Get Up and Go!

Body Fat: Friend and Foe
  Why Your Doctor Frowns If You Are Overfat
  What Do You Want to Lose?
  Swear Off the Scale
  *As the Fat Shrinks, Count Down the Inches

*Progress Evaluation

Get a Line on Labels
  *Pantry Inventory
  *Breakfast Bottles and Boxes

*Eating Diary

*Practice Diary One

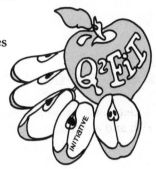

It's About Time

Although there may be a more convenient time, there really is no perfect time to have a baby, move to another city, change jobs, or stop smoking. There is likewise no optimum time to begin making changes toward a healthier lifestyle—unless you really *want* to change.

With each passing day, someone within earshot can be heard to say, "I need to get rid of some of this extra fat" or "I should get in shape—just look at me!" "Shoulds" and "oughtas" are not the same as "want tos"—which are still not the same as doing. Just compare the money spent on fitness togs, health clubs, and "diet" schemes with the number of people who are still overfat and out of shape.

Psychologists agree that continually complaining about one's health but not doing anything to improve it is unproductive; it fosters obsessive guilt while reinforcing a sense of powerlessness (i.e., "I haven't accomplished anything yet, so I guess I never will"). This attitude can lead to compulsive eating, chronic "dieting," and serious damage to self-image.

If you sincerely want to boost your health and appearance, on the other hand, nothing can stop you. Getting started is the toughest part—like pedaling a bicycle up a hill. Even a conditioned athlete would have to use the climbing gear at first, but the anticipation of the downhill ride helps to spur that initial push. If these lifestyle changes seem arduous right now, don't worry; very soon you get to lean back for the downhill coast.

Just because you aren't gung-ho at this moment doesn't mean the initiative is permanently out of your grasp. Weigh the costs versus the benefits of change. Rather than fretting about all of life's pleasures you will have to give up, consider cutting *down* rather than cutting *out*. As an alternative, you might develop positive passions like recreational sports or natural-foods cooking to replace less productive addictions. Pour your effort into doing rather than *not* doing. Seek the company of vivacious people who are engaged in the kinds of activities you'd like to take up—their vitality could be contagious. One accountant admits beginning a jogging program because "I was the only one in my office who didn't run, and I felt like the oddball."

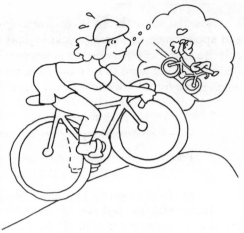

Envision the Downhill Coast

ARE YOU GAME FOR CHANGE?

List some immediate and long-term benefits you will enjoy by improving your health and appearance. Conjure up an image of the new and improved you.

> More energy
> Look better
> Clothes fit
> Self-esteem

If you pictured yourself healthy and happy, now list some activities you look forward to participating in as a healthier, happier person. Write down how you will look and feel doing them.

> Running on The beach

Jot down a few things that are likely to be stumbling blocks as you get your project rolling, such as holidays, houseguests, financial stress, bad weather, or the new baby. Circle the biggest obstacle and think of creative ways to deal with it.

Stumbling Blocks	Creative Solutions
Time	Learn to say no,
Entertaining Len	More exercise

Now list some things you will have to give up in order to improve your health and appearance or some psychological negatives that could make changes difficult. Be specific. ("No one cares anyway"; "I don't have time"; "I'm afraid of failing again"; "I don't want to give up steak and gravy"; "Am I worth this effort?"; "I'd be responsible for a 'new me'—can I cope?")

Large satisfying lunches
Wine
I don't have time

Reexamine this last list. Of those things that are precious to you, is it imperative they be forever banned? Or could you simply enjoy them less often? And when you weigh the disadvantages against the advantages of change, which comes out ahead? Your answer will help you decide whether you can honestly sign the following agreement.

PARTICIPATION AGREEMENT

Now, are you ready—really ready—to begin Living Lean? Then read the Participation Agreement through at least two times. If there are any statements you'd like to change, add, or delete, pencil in the alterations. Even though there's no fine print, this is a binding contract, so consider it thoughtfully before signing. Have a supportive person be your witness if possible.

I really *want* to lose fat and become fit.

I am solely responsible for my self-improvement project and will enlist the support of others when necessary.

I acknowledge this ongoing project as a current priority in my life.

I am comfortable with realistic, long-term goals consisting of positive thoughts and constructive actions, since they will produce the most enduring benefits.

I will make changes for the better in my lifestyle and habits because my health and happiness are important to me.

_____	_____
Signature	Date
_____	_____
Witness	Date

TREASURE MAPPING FOR SUCCESS

Do you really and truly want to be healthy and fit? Lean and happy? Whatever your goals for your Living Lean project, consider creating a Treasure Map to help you achieve them.

Here's what you do. Select a piece of paper in a color that appeals to you. Find a photo in a magazine or elsewhere that symbolizes the way you would like to look and, more important, the way you would like to *feel*. One woman, for example, had an artist friend sketch her with healthier contours. Now paste the picture on the paper, and with a bright-colored marker write your goal or heart's desire as a positive statement in the present tense: "I am poised and in control"; "I feel happy and energetic"; "I am confident and proud of my body." (No tentative statements like "I am getting better" are accepted; the Treasure Map goes for the gold—"I am *great*.")

You may hear voices from your subconscious arguing "No, it's not true" or "It can't happen" while you're writing your statement. Ignore this negative self, and start reprogramming with positive possibilities.

Keep your map handy—in a drawer, on your desk, in the kitchen or car— and look at it daily until you can see the picture in your mind's eye. Though the Treasure Map is simple and direct, you'll find it packs a more powerful punch than a traditional list of goals because of its visual reinforcement.

Does this technique really work? One woman discovered that her vision had become reality two years after she "forgot" about her Treasure Map, so give it plenty of time. If nothing else, it's easy, it's fun, it's positive, and it sets your ambitions in motion. For such a small investment, you have little to lose. Try it and see!

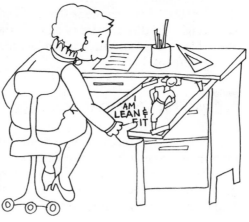

Make It Happen

Positively Speaking
(and Thinking and Doing)

Have you ever noticed that *successful* athletes, movie stars, or politicians rarely put themselves down? In this project, the primary competition will be the negative you, and the best way to take on your opponent is to recognize negativity when it occurs. It may be present in feelings, expressed in thoughts, or repressed into your subconscious. It's only natural to feel sorry for yourself or doubtful of your potential at times, but this is extremely unproductive.

Negative word associations can generate negative results, say Living Lean students, so they have compiled a list of words and phrases that have subtle but powerful negative connotations for them. The following are a few examples, and you may have others you'd like to add. (At one class we symbolically set fire to our list, but this is not recommended, as it tends to set off the smoke alarm.)

- on a diet
- free food
- take it off
- willpower

- goal weight
- counting calories
- binge
- reduce

- blubber
- forbidden
- cheat
- blow it

Be careful even when what you say or think is obviously true. "I am overfat" sounds as immutable as "They are wealthy" or "She is beautiful." However, the stock market can crash, age can mar beauty, and fat *can* be burned! If you keep repeating to yourself "I am so fat" day after day, you program your subconscious to continue acting on this image, which it mistakenly accepts as permanent. So cancel that thought and substitute a more productive one: "I have excess body fat right now, but it is decreasing"; or even better, "My body is growing more lean and healthy every day." Learn to say "I am more lean" instead of "I am less fat."

ACCENTUATE THE POSITIVE

Living Lean students almost unanimously agree that positive thoughts are a prerequisite for productive actions. To encourage positive thinking, try this technique when a negative thought drifts across your mind. Say "Cancel that thought" and replace it with a positive statement. For example:

"I can never resist chocolate cream pie."

"Cancel that thought. I don't have to eat a dessert every time it's available."

"I'm just not the athletic type."

"Cancel that thought. I'm out of shape now, but I'm determined to keep walking until I get in shape."

 ARE YOU A POSITIVE PERSON?

Test your positive thinking. Answer these questions as honestly as possible, using this scoring system: circle 5 for an answer of Always or Definitely; 4 for Usually; 3 for Sometimes; 2 for Rarely; and 1 for Never.

1. When the unexpected forces you to change your plans, are you quick to spot a hidden advantage in the new situation?   1 2 ③ 4 5

2. When you catch a stranger staring at you, do you assume it's because he or she finds you attractive?   1 2 ③ 4 5

3. Do you like most of the people you meet?   1 2 3 ④ 5

4. When you think about next year, do you tend to think you'll be better off than you are now?   1 2 3 4 ⑤

5. Do you often stop to admire things of beauty?   1 2 ③ 4 5

6. When someone finds fault with you or something you've done, can you tell the difference between constructive criticism and destructive criticism (which is best ignored)?   1 2 3 ④ 5

7. Do you praise your spouse, best friend, or child more often than you criticize him or her?   1 2 3 4 ⑤

8. Do you believe the human race will survive through the next century?   1 2 3 4 ⑤

9. Are you surprised when a friend lets you down?   1 2 3 ④ 5

10. Do you consider yourself a happy person?   1 2 3 ④ 5

11. If a police officer stopped you for speeding when you were quite certain you were not, would you firmly argue your case and even take it to court to prove you were right?   1 ② 3 4 5

12. Are you comfortable making jokes about yourself? Can you laugh at your imperfections? 1 2 3 4 5

13. Do you believe that, overall, your present state of mind has a positive effect on your physical health? 1 2 3 4 5

14. If you made a list of the ten people you admire most, could *your* name be on the list? 1 2 3 4 5

15. When you think back over the past few months, do you tend to remember your little successes more than your setbacks and failures? 1 2 3 4 5

Scoring:

If you scored 65 or more, consider yourself a "superstar"—someone whose optimism is a powerful, healing force.

60–65: Excellent—you're a genuine positive thinker.

55–60: Good—you're a positive thinker—sometimes.

50–55: Fair—your positive side and your negative side are about evenly matched.

50 and below: Do you see any consistent negative patterns? Where could you improve?

From *Complete Guide to Your Emotions*, copyright 1986 by Rodale Press, Inc. Reprinted by permission of Rodale Press, Inc., Emmaus, Pa.

Medical Exam and Personal Health Record

If you do not already have a physician who counsels you on the importance of eating healthy and staying physically active, then find one. In addition, keep a folder containing personal health records and medical history for each family member. You can assume this information is contained in your various physicians' files, but you can't be assured it will be readily available in an emergency. Know your usual blood pressure, blood lipids, medications—including how much you take and how often—immunizations, and any other vital statistics. Your health is *your* responsibility, not your physician's.

Advise your doctor that you will be increasing your physical activity and altering your diet to include more fiber and less fat. If you are more than 35 years old or in very poor physical condition, your doctor will probably suggest a physical and laboratory exam and possibly an exercise stress test before you begin the changes. Request a blood lipid profile, including HDL-cholesterol and relevant ratios. These provide valid information about your risk of cardiovascular disease and will help you plan your aerobic activities accordingly. Also, your medication requirement for diabetes or hypertension treatment may decrease during the Living Lean project, so your blood sugar or blood pressure should be monitored closely until they stabilize.

The dietary suggestions in this book are compatible with most prescribed diets, but occasionally a special problem—like an allergy to dairy products—will require individual attention from your professional nutritionist.

In general, the entire family will benefit from the healthful changes explained in *Living Lean by Choosing More*, so there's no need to fix separate meals for each person. Be honest but subtle in presenting new foods, though. "It's good for you" rarely sells; good food that tastes good is always a hit. Remember, there's no need to rush—productive changes take time.

One final caution: skimping on protein or calories is *not* recommended for growing children, pregnant or nursing women, family members recovering from illness, the elderly, or anyone in poor health. The same goes for those engaged in heavy physical labor or intensive training programs. If questions arise, don't hesitate to ask your physician and nutritionist for answers.

✏ GET UP AND GO!

Did you get your medical clearance? Great—now plunge right in. Start by taking a short walk *now*. (Or if it's too late today, then first thing tomorrow.) Sure, the weather may be less than perfect, but you can bundle up or wait until the cool of evening to venture out. You are physically hardier than you think. Spending your entire life behind closed doors will not train your body to adjust to changes.

If there is absolutely no convenient or comfortable place for you to walk (park, stadium, shopping mall, office building, beach) or if you are physically unable to walk, then you are face to face with a key obstacle to your health and fitness project. (You'll get some ideas for overcoming fitness obstacles in Chapter 5.) There is always (yes, *always*) a solution. Write down some alternative possibilities because, where body fat is concerned, if you *move* it, you'll *lose* it.

Safe and Convenient Places Where I Can Walk

Body Fat: Friend and Foe

Have you ever wondered why your body goes to such extremes to store fat you don't want? One reason is that your body fat protects against mechanical injury. Another reason is that it acts as a heat insulator. Fat added during pregnancy is an energy reserve for the nursing mother, a reserve that may be depleted *only* with extended breastfeeding.

Even more important than these reasons is simple survival. Our ancestors' bodies were adept at storing fat in anticipation of constant famines. For them, it was survival of the *fattest*. Although this is still true for some people in some areas of the world, for most of us famine means "I didn't have time to eat today." When you reach the bottom line, your excess fat is more likely to be a health liability than survival insurance.

WHY YOUR DOCTOR FROWNS IF YOU ARE OVERFAT

A patient limps painfully into the doctor's office and moans, "Doc, my arthritis is acting up something terrible."

"We're going to have to work on this extra fat you're backpacking," the doctor replies.

"I realize that, Doc, but what I'm concerned about right now is this hip. The pain is unbearable."

"You've got to get your body weight down," says the doctor firmly.

The patient, still confused, thinks he and the physician are experiencing a communication breakdown. But the physician knows the burden of excess body fat places a strain on weight-bearing joints. Treating the hip merely eliminates a symptom of the true problem.

In addition to joint stress, people who are too heavy also have a greater risk of diabetes; renal disease and kidney stones; cardiovascular disease, including hypertension, stroke, and elevated blood lipids; gall bladder disease; gout; lung disease; breast and endometrial cancer, menstrual irregularities, sterility, and toxemia of pregnancy. Other side effects include breathing difficulties like snoring, flat feet, infections in skin folds, organ compression, varicose veins, and poor heat tolerance. Those who have excessive body fat are usually out of shape and may not be able to rely on their bodies to perform optimally in an emergency. They are poor surgical risks and they also die at an earlier age.

WHAT DO YOU WANT TO LOSE?

For medical reasons and more, everyone wants to lose weight these days. But losing weight is not necessarily a guarantee of losing body fat. To an announcement of "Guess what? I lost 10 pounds last week," *Fit or Fat?* author Covert Bailey has a clever retort: "Pounds of what?" A rapid weight loss or gain—say, 4 pounds between Friday night and Monday morning—indicates something in addition to fat has disappeared.

It could be water. Since your body is about 60 percent water, fluctuations in body fluids can show up on the scale as a sizable number of pounds. Or it could be glycogen. This energy reserve—weighing more than a pound—will shrink over the course of a day if you fail to eat enough carbohydrate or if you (ahem) "forget" to eat. You later bounce on the scale with glee because you have "lost weight." But hold the hoorays because it isn't only fat that has vanished. Glycogen and its associated water (totaling 3 or 4 pounds) and even some body protein have disappeared as well.

The next day or so you experience an imperceptible increase in appetite as your body restores this naturally occurring fuel reserve, along with its accompanying water. You step on the scale again and . . . drat—a weight *gain*. Through all these dramatic weight changes there may be *no substantial change in body fat*.

Wouldn't an intentional, well-planned, low-calorie diet produce better results? Not at first. Each pound of glycogen has about 3 to 4 pounds of water packaged with it when it's put in storage. During the first few days of a 1,000-calorie diet, mostly glycogen reserves are burned for energy, and again a couple of pounds of associated water disappear along with it. (A little muscle protein is also sacrificed, along with *its* associated water.)

When volunteers in one study were put on an actual 1,000-calorie diet, the first several days' weight loss was 70 percent water and 5 percent lean muscle. In other words, of 4 pounds lost, 3 were not fat. So much for "The Fabulous Four-Pound Weekend Diet." Thus, cutting calories for just a few days can produce an impressive initial weight loss (mostly water and glycogen), and the dieter is hopelessly hooked.

When the "diet" finally ends and the table is again set with a reasonable amount of food and adequate carbohydrate, the glycogen and water will be fully replaced, just as they should be. In one study, 5½ scale-pounds were added in only four days—of which 4½ pounds were water. Even with no change in calories, health status, or activity, normal people can experience glycogen or water weight shifts of up to 2 pounds per day. All of this means that "pounds" are more meaningful when you are on a splendid shopping spree in London.

Part of the problem here is that burning real fat—like burning a big oak log—is slow going. It's difficult to ignite, but once it catches fire it provides steady heat for a long time. Thus, body fat is a key to endurance energy. Glycogen, a carbohydrate, provides a more immediate fuel source, as when you sprint to catch the bus. Like kindling twigs, it's easy to ignite but rather short-lived, providing a quick burst of energy. A combination of the two fuels is more effective than either one alone since they work as a team. (Unfortunately, overfat folks often have proportionately more fat-storing hormones than fat-releasing hormones, so they may have trouble mobilizing fat fuel efficiently during exertion. Consistent training helps to correct that imbalance.)

Weight loss, then, can be quick and easy. But real fat loss *must* be slow. Except for a very large person or someone shedding a lot of water, 1 scale-pound a week is a maximum weight loss, and ½ pound a week may be an optimum—both to protect health and to ensure that positive changes in body composition and body image are permanent.

SWEAR OFF THE SCALE

What does the scale register when you step on it? *All* your body parts—skeleton, organs, glycogen, water, and muscle—not just fat. Most of these components (except perhaps glycogen and water) don't fluctuate much from day to day, and that includes your body fat.

This means two people could weigh the same, yet one could be very lean, like a body builder, and the other could be overfat, like an armchair athlete. (An overweight person could also retain water or have dense, heavy bones, both of which show up on the scale as extra pounds.) Professional football players exemplify big guys who don't fit the height and weight tables. They are overweight by these standards, but there is hardly any excess fat on them. On one professional football team, the average body fat ratio is 11 percent—only 22 fat-pounds out of 200.

Quite the contrast is a woman in her late forties whose weight is the same as it was in high school. She doesn't realize her lean tissue—mainly unused muscle—has gradually and insidiously shrunk, while her fat layer has expanded in its place. (The average person gains a pound of fat each year after age 25. He or she also loses a fourth to a half pound of lean each year, resulting in additional fat replacing the lost muscle. A gain of 30 scale-pounds by age 55 could mean an actual increase of 45 fat-pounds!)

Even when you are making healthy progress, the scale may indicate the opposite: trading fat for muscle when you begin an aerobic activity routine can register as a slight increase in pounds the first few weeks. The more out of shape you are, the longer it takes to replace those muscles you should never have lost. For Living Lean purposes, height and weight charts can be misleading and the bathroom scale downright deceiving. Since many "professional dieters" also harbor negative feelings toward the scale, you are encouraged *not to weigh*.

If weight is such an unreliable yardstick, how do you go about determining how much body fat you have? More important, how do you measure changes—let's hope they're decreases—in that fat? For a precise body composition analysis, clinicians use underwater weight, electronic counters, or bioelectrical impedance measures.

The caliper pinch test is a fair approximation and is now used routinely by many physicians and professional nutritionists. Just one warning: don't try to compare values derived from one technique with those from another. And if you can pinch an inch-thick fold of fat on the back of your upper arm, you've got too much fat.

For a rough estimate of your body fat percentage, you might use the Body Fat Indicator Scale (Appendix A). But if you have a strong hunch there's too much fat on your frame, knowing the precise amount of fat isn't as helpful as being able to monitor before-and-after changes in fat.

HOW MUCH FAT IS TOO MUCH FAT?

Females generally carry more body fat than males—and they are supposed to. Specifically, more than 30 percent body fat (for a woman) or 25 percent fat (for a man) would be considered overfat. (If you weigh 100 pounds, 20 percent body fat is equivalent to 20 pounds of fat.) A desirable percentage of body fat might be 15 to 20 percent for a man and 20 to 28 percent for a woman. Conditioned, competing athletes often carry even less fat than normal, lean individuals.

Please note, there is no "ideal" body fat percentage. The limits given here are only tentative, and some folks are no doubt healthier at a higher percentage within these suggested ranges.

AS THE FAT SHRINKS, COUNT DOWN THE INCHES

A simple at-home technique will help you quantify your progress. Since the change in subcutaneous fat (the layer of fat under your skin) usually reflects the change in your total body fat, you can keep tabs by monitoring the pluses and minuses in your girth measurements. In other words, stop counting down the pounds, and start counting down the inches.

Using a cloth tape measure (the dime store should have one), measure and record each circumference as indicated. Enlist the aid of a friend or family member if you like; it will help validate your improvements if you have a witness—especially if he or she is generous with supportive compliments.

	Beginning of Project	After Eight Weeks	Follow-up
Bust or chest (widest point)	_____	_____	_____
Waist (one inch above belly button)	_____	_____	_____
Hips (widest point)	_____	_____	_____
Upper arm (midway between shoulder and elbow)	_____	_____	_____
Forearm (widest point)	_____	_____	_____
Thigh (just below buttocks)	_____	_____	_____
Calf (widest mid-point)	_____	_____	_____

There is no "ideal" bust, chest, or thigh measurement, thank goodness. Instead, watch for decreases, which will become evident when the waistband of your favorite skirt or pair of slacks ceases to strangle your middle, and you are able to take a deep breath in a flattering, expensive suit.

Now look closely at your waist, chest, and hip measurements—they are important health-risk indicators. For each inch your waist exceeds your chest, you lose two years in the game of life expectancy.

waist measurement − chest measurement = _____ × 2 = _____

Next, divide your waist measurement by your hip measurement. If the quotient is larger than 0.8 (for a woman) or 1.0 (for a man), your risk of stroke, heart disease, diabetes, hypertension, and elevated triglycerides increases. In fact, the leanest men with the biggest bellies may incur the greatest risk. If you're Living Lean, it pays to be a *waist* watcher, not a weight watcher.

waist measurement ÷ hip measurement = _____

BODY BEAUTIFUL

Of 60 modern cultures, only seven (including ours) place any value on thinness. Regardless of our own sentiments or of high-fashion society, "girl fat" (the padded thighs, the rounded hips) is natural, and it is not unhealthy. It's supposed to be there to provide enough calories to nourish a baby before and after birth. On the other hand, "boy fat" (the belt overhang, the spare tire) is a health liability. It's not supposed to be there—on a man or on a woman.

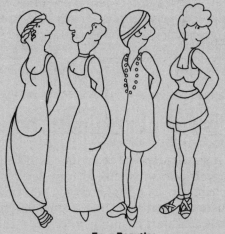

Four Beauties

Yet men are generally satisfied with their "love handles" (though women prefer them leaner) while women are generally dissatisfied with their own hips and thighs (though men may think they are just right). In other words, men ignore fat that could imperil their health while women abhor fat that is innocent of wrongdoing.

"Women will do anything to make themselves more beautiful," observe Living Lean students. But even the definition of beauty has changed substantially through history—from the swollen belly of fertility to the big-bustled behind, from the flat-chested flapper to the curvaceous calendar girl. And it wasn't too long ago that "well built" referred to a woman's big bust rather than her shapely quadriceps!

You might take time to ponder what "attractive" means to you. Pinpoint specific characteristics. Think of some people you know who fit the description. Do they also fit the Hollywood stereotype of handsome or beautiful? Do you think being healthy or physically fit makes people look better? Do you think becoming more attractive is within your grasp?

✏️ Progress Evaluation

"How am I doing? Am I making progress? If not, am I at least maintaining any previous improvements?" Here are some important signals of progress for you to monitor. You may want to add some criteria of your own. Evaluate yourself at the beginning of the project and again after eight weeks, at the end of the project. Try not to peek in the meantime. (Remember, look for effort and improvement rather than perfection.) Then evaluate again as often as necessary in the future.

This week, rate yourself on each item. Put an **X** on the line at a point that represents your current status. ("Waist measurement" and "snug-fitting skirt or slacks" are already marked to help you get started.) After eight weeks, reevaluate with a star (*) on each line. Later, you can use a check mark (✓) for your first follow-up.

Waist measurement	increased ———— X ————	decreased
Snug-fitting skirt or slacks	snugger ———— X ————	looser
Lean-to-fat body composition (Appendix A)	overfat ———— X ————	very lean
Fitness level (Appendix B)	very poor ———— X ————	very good
Energy level	very poor —— X ————	very good
Sleep quality	very poor —— X ————	very good
Self-appreciation	very poor —— X ————	very good
Overall mood	very poor ———— X ————	very good
Related health problems:		
Blood pressure	too high/too low ———— X — normal (90–120/60–80 mm Hg)	
Blood cholesterol	too high/too low ———— X — normal (120–200 mg/100 ml)	
Blood glucose (fasting)	too high/too low ———— X normal (70–110 mg/100 ml)	
Realistic, patient attitude toward Living Lean project	rarely ———— X ————	almost always
Other:	worse ————————	better
	worse ————————	better

Get a Line on Labels

"Two ounces of tuna supply a fourth of your daily requirement for protein and vitamin B_{12}, and a substantial amount of niacin and vitamin B_6. Out of 60 calories, the fat content is less than a gram—that's low. This particular product is packed in spring water and vegetable broth, and salt is also added. For only a 2-ounce serving, the sodium content is 310 milligrams—and that's high." This dietitian friend who conducts supermarket tours appears to be a walking encyclopedia when it comes to food facts. Her secret? "If customers ask about an item, I take it off the shelf and read the entire label, right on the spot."

The label may not tell you everything you want to know, but it does tell you a lot that you need to know—*if* you read it. If you're not into nutritional analysis, simply examine the fine print after the word "ingredients"—it's much more informative than the splashy advertising claims on the front of the package. You might ask yourself the following questions before you toss the product into your shopping cart:

- Which ingredients are listed first? (Ingredients appear in relative order by weight, ranging from most to least. You still have to guess at the absolute amount of each ingredient, though.)
- Do the ingredients sound familiar? Would you use them in your kitchen? (One high-fiber bread was enriched with nonnutritive fiber, the equivalent of ordinary sawdust.)
- Are the ingredients wholesome and nutritious? (Salt and sugar make foods taste good, but as immoderate additives, they are nutritional negatives.)

It's up to you to fight label illiteracy—read your labels! Throughout this book, look for more Label Lingo suggestions.

LABEL LINGO

To tell the truth, labels can be pretty misleading when it comes to salt and sugar.

- "No sugar added" or "sugar-free" products could still contain honey, fructose, corn syrup, or another sweetener.
- "No salt added," "unsalted," or "low-salt" products could still be high in natural sodium or sodium additives.
- "Reduced sodium" products have 75 percent less sodium than usual, but they could still be very high in sodium.
- Don't despair—you're generally safe with terms like "low sodium" (less than 140 milligrams per serving), "very low sodium" (less than 35 milligrams per serving), "sodium-free," or "no refined sweeteners added."

PANTRY INVENTORY

Here is a task that will reacquaint you with the foods you think are already familiar. Choose a time when you and an interested accomplice—perhaps a family member—can operate as a team (getting others involved in your project can have numerous benefits).

One person scrutinizes each can, jar, bottle, and bag in the refrigerator, in the pantry, and especially in the spice cabinet. The other person lists all foods that contain added sodium or sugar and where each appears on the ingredient label. Don't overlook sugar twins like dextrose, sorbitol, xylitol, and "yeast food." For example:

Food	Sugar	Sodium
Honey-granola bread	3, 4, 6	8, 12

This bread contains honey, listed third; corn syrup, listed fourth; and raisin syrup, listed sixth. (Manufacturers use a combination of sweeteners so that sugar doesn't appear to be a major ingredient.) It also contains salt, eighth; and a sodium preservative, twelfth.

YOUR INVENTORY

Food	Sugar	Sodium

BREAKFAST BOTTLES AND BOXES

These are typical ingredient labels you would find on common breakfast items. See if you can identify them before looking at the list of choices. If not, try matching each breakfast food with its ingredient label.

_____ Enriched wheat flour, strawberry filling (corn syrup, dextrose, strawberries, crackermeal, apples, wheat starch, partially hydrogenated soybean oil, citric acid, color), partially hydrogenated soybean oil, corn syrup, sugar, whey, dextrose, salt, baking powder, baking soda, vitamins, iron.

_____ Water, corn syrup, partially hydrogenated soybean oil, mono- and diglycerides, soy protein, sodium stearoyl lactylate, polysorbate 60, dipotassium phosphate, disodium phosphate, sodium acid pyrophosphate, artificial flavor and color.

_____ Sugar, malted milk, nonfat dry milk, sodium caseinate, cocoa, maltodextrin, isolated soy protein, sweet dairy whey, lactose, calcium caseinate, magnesium hydroxide, artificial vanilla flavors, lecithin, carageenan, sodium ascorbate (vitamin C), salt, other vitamins, iron.

_____ Milk, chocolate (sugar, cocoa butter, whole milk powder, chocolate liquor, lecithin, salt, vanillin), crisp rice (rice, sugar, salt, malt), peanut butter (peanuts, sucrose, hydrogenated vegetable oil [cottonseed and/or rapeseed and/or palm oil], salt), invert sugar, rolled oats, peanuts, corn syrup, brown sugar, corn syrup solids, rolled whole wheat, honey, glycerin, partially hydrogenated vegetable oil (soybean and/or palm and/or cottonseed oil), nonfat milk, dried unsweetened coconut, almonds, salt, natural and artificial flavors, BHA (a preservative), citric acid (a stabilizing agent).

_____ Water, high-fructose corn syrup, concentrated orange juice, sugar, concentrated lemon juice, orange pulp, natural flavors, concentrated grapefruit, tangerine, and lime juices.

_____ Rolled oats, sugar, creaming agent (maltodextrin, partially hydrogenated coconut oil, sodium caseinate, dipotassium phosphate, mono- and diglycerides, sodium silicoaluminate, artificial flavor, riboflavin), flavored fruit pieces (dehydrated apples treated with sulfur dioxide, sodium sulfite, and sodium bisulfite), dehydrated peaches, artificial flavor, citric acid, annatto color, salt, calcium carbonate, guar gum, artificial flavor, vitamins, iron.

_____ 100 percent rolled oats with oat bran.

_____ Partially hydrogenated and liquid soybean oil, water, salt, whey, sodium benzoate (a preservative), lecithin, artificial flavor, vitamin A palmitate, beta carotene (color).

A. nondairy creamer
B. peanut butter granola bar
C. frozen concentrated citrus beverage
D. margarine

E. instant breakfast shake
F. strawberry toaster pastry
G. peach-flavored instant oatmeal
H. quick-cooking oatmeal

Answers: F, A, E, B, C, G, H, D

✐ Eating Diary

Before choosing the appropriate route for a cross-country trip, you need to decide what your departure point will be and then have your auto checked out for any problems that need attention. In the same way, to effect changes in what and how you eat, it's important to do some consciousness-raising about your current eating habits. Some practices may need only minor repairs, while others demand an extensive overhaul, but the mechanical work will facilitate the journey from where you are to where you want to be.

The best way to know exactly what you eat is to write it all down. Record right now (yes, take a few minutes)—regardless of whether it has been a good or bad day, whether it's morning or late at night—*everything* you have eaten or drunk so far today. Complete today's record. Then log your oral travels for two more days.

Use the Eating Diary form if you wish. It will provide extra information that could come in handy: why you eat, when you eat, where you eat, and so on. In addition, you may want to record a weekend day, since your usual routine is often disrupted after the five o'clock whistle on Friday. Suggestion: don't plan ahead for this activity. You may be tempted to alter your accustomed eating pattern, and this is one diary that should "tell it like it is!"

✐ ✓ Practice Diary One

Even doing something an easier way seems like more trouble at first because it's a *different* way. When making changes in your habits, think evolution, not revolution. It takes at least three weeks to make or break a habit, so don't give up after two and a half. The nice thing about new habits is that they will become as entrenched and resistant to change as the old ones if you simply practice them enough.

That's where the Practice Diary comes in. Check off (✓) activities like the Pantry Inventory and Medical Exam as you complete them, and don't forget to record your measurements so you can enjoy watching them shrink. For ongoing practices like your Eating Diary, check off each day you make an effort to work on them. Include any helpful information on your Practice Diary, then keep it handy so you can use it.

If any of the Suggested Practices appeal to you, add them to your main practice list. Or just check them off as you work on them. If you need more than a week of effort on any practice (which *is* a possibility), extend it to the following week's Practice Diary. Investing more time and effort just might pay off; old habits die hard, but we have living, breathing testimony that they do die. *Think evolution, not revolution.*

EATING DIARY

Time/how long	Food or drink and amount	Fried, greasy, or hidden fat (✓)	Where eaten/ while doing what	Alone or with company	Why eaten/mood	Hunger rating (1 to 5)

Time/how long: note the time of each meal and snack and how long it took to eat.

Food or drink and amount: include alcohol, sugar-free sodas, sugar in coffee, butter on toast, even water if you like; use a scale or measuring cups and spoons at first, or estimate the amount.

Fried, greasy, or hidden fat: put a check mark (✓) if yes.

Where eaten/while doing what: note the specific place, like kitchen table, car, couch, and any activities, such as watching TV, talking on phone, reading paper.

Alone or with company: indicate with an A or a C; or you can note who the company is—your toddler, the Happy Hour gang, your family.

Why eaten/mood: jot down why you ate—ravenous, skipped breakfast, everyone else eating, food commercial on TV; or describe your mood—bored, angry, nervous, elated, fatigued.

Hunger rating: rank your hunger *before* eating on a scale of 1 to 5; 1 would be "uncomfortably full" and 5 would be "overhungry."

RECORD MEALS AND SNACKS

SUNDAY

MONDAY

TUESDAY

WEDNESDAY

THURSDAY

FRIDAY

SATURDAY

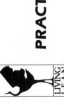

PRACTICE DIARY ONE

Practices

Practices	Su	M	Tu	W	Th	F	Sa	Notes
Medical Exam								
Count Down the Inches								
Progress Evaluation								
Pantry Inventory								
Eating Diary								

✓ = yes, I did try;   ✓✓ = yes, I did welll

Suggested Practices

- Are You Game for Change? List expected personal benefits from your Living Lean project, both immediate and lasting.
- Creat a Treasure Map and look at it daily.
- Accentuate the Positive. Cancel negative thought dialogues and replace them with positive ones.
- Get Up and Go! Locate convenient places to walk and begin walking.
- Swear Off the Scale.

WEEK TWO

What's the Verdict? Eating Diary Analysis
   *Eating Habits Checkup
   *Nutrition Checkup

The Fiber Connection: Filling, Not Fattening
   Fiber: Good for What Ails You
   Outstanding Fiber Foods
   Shopping with Fiber in Mind
   Practice: Focus on Fiber

Tame Your Appetite
   Set the Timing: Graze, Don't Gorge
   Eat Often (and You'll Eat Less)
   Snappy Snacks
   Practice: Fill in the Snack Gaps

The Caffeine Scene
   Practice: Taper Off Mr. Caffeine

*Practice Diary Two

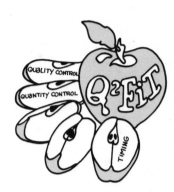

What's the Verdict? Eating Diary Analysis

Once you become aware of your unproductive eating habits, you can pay special attention to them when they are discussed in the coming chapters. Look over your Eating Diary and check (✓) any of the following statements that seem to apply. Put double checks (✓✓) by those that are a definite "yes." Then, if you want, go back through and briefly answer the questions after each statement you checked. Be as specific as possible: "drank sodas while watching TV in the evening," "ate fast-food taco due to early-morning meeting," or "angry at spouse, led to milkshake."

EATING HABITS CHECKUP

Time

_____ More than four hours between meals/snacks (Which ones? How many hours? Why?)

_____ Mealtimes erratic, skipped; insubstantial meals (Which ones? How often? Why?)

_____ Snacks but no regular meals (How often? Why?)

_____ Late or extra-large supper (How often? Why?)

_____ Heavy snacks after supper (What foods? How often? Why?)

_____ Most of calories late in day (How often? Why?)

How Long

_____ Finished meal in less than 20 minutes (Which meal? What situation or why?)

_____ Gulped down snack food or drink (What food? What time? What situation or why?)

Food and Amount

_____ Alcohol (Number of drinks per day or week? What kind? What time or which meal? Where or what situation?)

_____ Caffeine drinks (Number of cups or cans of regular coffee, tea, soft drinks, or sugar-free drinks per day or week? What time or which meal? Where or what situation?)

_____ Soft drinks (Number of drinks per day or week? What kind? What time or which meal? Where or what situation?)

_____ Sweets, pastry, candy, and desserts (What foods? How much? What time or which meal? Where or what situation? How often?)

_____ Chips and processed snack foods (What foods? What time or which meal? Where or what situation? How often?)

_____ Salty foods other than above—ham, canned soup, Oriental food (What foods? What time or which meal? How often?)

_____ Greasy, fatty, or fried foods—cheese, nuts, sausage (What foods? What time or which meal? Where or what situation? How often?)

_____ Added fats—butter, salad dressing, mayonnaise (What foods? How much? How often?)

_____ Convenience foods—canned, processed, frozen dinners (What foods? What time or which meal? How often?)

_____ Little variety (What foods repeated or missing? Which meal or snack? Why?)

_____ Too much of certain foods (What foods? How much? What time or which meal?)

Where Eaten

_____ More meals out (How many per week? Which meals? Favorite types of restaurants?)

_____ More meals at home (How many per week? Which meals? Are meals out or meals at home more nutritious? Why?)

_____ Meals other than at the table (Which meals? Where?)

_____ Snacks other than at the table (What foods? What time? Where?)

Alone or with Company

_____ More meals alone (Which meals?)

_____ More meals with company (Which meals? Are meals alone or meals with company more nutritious? Why?)

Situation or Mood

_____ Eating for reasons other than hunger (What foods? What time? While doing what? What situation or why? What mood?)

_____ Binge eating (What foods? What time? What situation or why? What mood?)

_____ Nibbling or picking at food (What foods? What time? While doing what? What situation or why? What mood?)

Hunger

_____ Overhungry (What time? Why?)

_____ Not hungry for meal (What time or which meal? Why?)

Now complete the Nutrition Checkup on the following page.

In the Your Daily Servings column which total comes out ahead—high-fiber, nutrient-dense, less processed foods (on the left), or lower-fiber, calorie-dense, more processed foods (on the right)? Did you eat at least the minimum number of recommended servings for the various food groups? Based on your Nutrition Checkup and your Eating Habits Checkup, summarize any eating problems that could hinder your Living Lean project. For example, consider how often, how much, and how fast you eat as well as how your mood or social setting influences your eating habits.

What _specific_ changes would help correct the problem in each category?

A hearty appetite signals good health, as any child's mother will attest. However, if your Eating Diary is fairly bursting at the seams, don't wrestle with willpower or struggle with starvation diets when _Living Lean by Choosing More_ has better ideas. The simple techniques described in this chapter can help you lasso your appetite _before_ it has a chance to run wild.

The Fiber Connection: Filling, Not Fattening

There's no arguing with your appetite after a long day of cleaning out the attic or hiking the nature trails; you will and should be hungry, and it appears fairly easy to overeat.

✎ NUTRITION CHECKUP

For this part of the analysis, look at your Eating Diary and write down the average number of servings you ate from each food group in a day. A rough estimate is fine. Typical serving sizes and recommended minimum number of servings are listed.

Food Group	Serving Size	Recommended Daily Servings	Your Daily Servings
GRAINS AND STARCHES Whole grains—bread, cereal, pasta, rice; starchy vegetables—corn, peas, potatoes, winter squash Refined white flour products	1 piece, ½ cup cooked	minimum 5 servings	____
LEGUME PROTEIN Dried beans—pinto beans, black-eyed peas, split peas; tofu	½ cup cooked, 4 ounces	serve often	____
ANIMAL PROTEIN Meat, cheese, cottage cheese, eggs (if less than 8 servings)	1 ounce meat or cheese	minimum 3 servings (women)	____
Meat, cheese, cottage cheese, eggs (if 8 servings or more)	¼ cup cottage cheese, 1 egg	or 4 servings (men)	
VEGETABLES Fresh or frozen, lightly cooked or raw vegetables Canned or boiled vegetables	½ cup cooked, 1 cup raw	minimum 3 servings	____
FRUIT Fresh, frozen unsweetened, or dried fruit Canned or sugar-added fruit	1 piece, ½ cup, ¼ cup dried	minimum 2 servings	____
MILK Skim or low-fat milk or yogurt Whole or 2½% milk or yogurt	1 cup	2 servings	____
		Totals	____

But exactly how much food is too much food? A small slice of strawberry pie is more than a gallon of salad if calories are the yardstick. And if you crowd the dinner table or fill your stomach, it doesn't necessarily mean you have abandoned Quantity Control because dietary fiber casts the deciding vote. For example, an apple may seem like a lot of food (and a more satisfying snack) when compared with a half cup of apple juice. But the calories are just the same—the only difference is fiber. And eating more high-fiber, high-volume, low-fat foods is a slick trick because it could cut your calories in *half*.

In a University of Alabama study, a low-to-high-fiber switch slashed participants' calories from 3,000 to 1,570 a day, even when they ate all they wanted. The fiber-full meals were rated just as tasty and filling, and didn't trigger extra nibbling to replace the saved calories. On the contrary, the low-fiber meals tended to induce overeating: participants failed to stop eating when they were pleasantly full.

Here are two typical menus tested in the study:

High-Fiber, Low-Calorie	Low-Fiber, High-Calorie
Orange slices	Orange juice
Oatmeal and bananas	Fried egg and bacon
Whole wheat toast with poached egg	Grits, white toast with margarine
Skim milk, coffee	Whole milk, coffee
Large chef salad with cheese and dressing	Ham with cheese, tomato, and bun
Rye crisp bread	French fries
Fresh fruit, tea	Baked beans, condiments
	Lemon pie, Coke
Baked chicken with brown rice pilaf	Roast beef, creamed potatoes with gravy
Broccoli with almonds	Green bean casserole
Lettuce with sliced tomatoes	Tossed salad with dressing
Fresh fruit	White roll with margarine
Whole wheat roll, tea	Chocolate cake, whole milk, tea

Even if your high-fiber experiment skims just 250 calories from your daily total instead of 1,430, that's an easy 2 fat-pounds lost in a month. Also, with some fiber foods you don't keep all the calories you eat. A USDA study found one month of extra fruits and veggies canceled 5 percent of the daily calories consumed by a group of middle-aged men. That is, 144 calories were never absorbed, and of those, 90 were fat calories. Dietary fiber evidently causes fat interference—and that's good. Bread and pasta lovers will be happy to hear that 2 to 10 percent of legitimate whole wheat calories are not absorbed, either. If you make some simple grocery list substitutions to include more fiber-rich foods, you should be able to write off 50 out of every 2,000 daily calories—a figure worth 5 fewer fat-pounds in a year's time.

It appears eating more dietary fiber is the easiest way to fight hunger and also maintain Quantity Control—*without* the hassle of counting calories. And if you've been avoiding carbohydrates because they are fattening, please hear this: fiber foods (all of them carbos) are filling, *not* fattening.

FIBER: GOOD FOR WHAT AILS YOU

Long ago, and not that far away, beans, biscuits, bread, and porridge were considered standard, hearty fare. Time passed, and poor folks' beans were traded for rich man's meat. Bread became pale to the point of sallow, and porridge gave way to talking puffed cereals.

Luckily we discovered our dreadful mistake before it was too late. Now fiber is the buzzword, and it means breakfast bran, not laundry lint. Lowly beans and grains are back on the menu, too, only this time they are presented as haute cuisine. In fact, these same foods that saved you money during the Depression era may well now save your health. You might never hear "take two burritos and call me in the morning," but old-fashioned, high-fiber eating benefits so many chronic and costly diseases it should be called the universal nutrition prescription.

Dietary fiber is good for much of what ails your digestive tract. Mechanically, it speeds up elimination and adds bulk, helping prevent constipation, varicose veins, hemorrhoids, hiatal hernia, diverticulitis, irritable colon, appendicitis, gall bladder disease, and even colon cancer in the process. Wheat bran is a high-performer in this category, and it's not habit-forming like some laxatives. Water-soluble fibers, on the other hand, bind with fats like cholesterol and carry them out of the body along with nasty carcinogens, reducing your risk of heart disease and, again, colon cancer. High-fiber diets have also been used in the treatment of diabetes and hypertension. Oat bran, dried beans, and apple pectin are especially effective.

But that's not all. Fiber holds food in your stomach longer, slowing down calorie absorption, preventing a rapid rise in blood sugar, and staving off hunger a little longer. Dried beans shine in this category, especially if they are presoaked and well cooked to release the soluble fiber. But there are other excellent choices, including oats, buckwheat, pasta, peas, sweet potatoes, corn, apples (instead of apple juice), oranges, and wheat bran.

Even if you eat less of your high-fiber foods, you still soak up more nutrients. White flour contains only 13 percent of the fiber in whole wheat, one-third as much chromium, one-fifth the zinc and magnesium, and only one-tenth the manganese. One researcher commented that a slice of white bread is nutritionally equivalent to a piece of bread concocted from 25 percent whole wheat flour and 75 percent sugar. That doesn't say much for the nutritional power of refined flour, but it says a lot in favor of fiber for Quality Control.

OUTSTANDING FIBER FOODS

Where do you get this all-purpose, lean-loving fiber? The ads on television would have you believe a bowl of bran-fortified cereal at breakfast and an occasional slice of whole wheat toast are all you need from the fiber department. But pioneering studies by Dr. Denis Burkitt in Africa found that a wide assortment of fiber foods—not a magical fiber supplement like bran—were responsible for better health, decreased degenerative disease, and greater longevity.

If you get confused and find yourself wondering, "What am I supposed to eat?" here are your staples—high in fiber, vitamins, and minerals and (except for nuts and seeds) low in fat—the backbone of Living Lean:

Dried beans and peas: 8 grams per serving (3/4 cup)
Pinto, black, red, white, kidney, navy, adzuki, garbanzo, and black-eyed peas and beans; lentils and split peas; soybeans, soy flour, soy grits, tofu, meat analogs

Whole grains: 2 to 4 grams per serving
100% whole wheat (bread, crackers, flour, cereal, pasta, tabouli, bulghur, tortillas); 100% whole rye (bread, crackers, flour, cooked cereal); corn (tortillas, cornmeal, corn bread, popcorn); oats (bran, flour, old-fashioned oatmeal, granola); brown rice (wild rice, flour, puffed rice cakes, crackers); buckwheat (pancakes, pasta, cereal groats, flour); millet (puffed cereal, flour); barley (pearled, flour); quinoa (cereal, flour); amaranth (cereal, flour)

Vegetables: 2 grams per serving

All, including green peas, lima beans, sweet potatoes, baked potatoes, corn, mixed vegetables, broccoli, green beans, okra, winter squash, artichokes, spinach, pumpkin, carrots, collard greens, tomatoes, and cabbage

Fruits: 2 grams per serving

All, including blackberries, raspberries, pears, apples, unsweetened applesauce, bananas, nectarines, oranges, peaches, papayas, strawberries, and dried fruit

Nuts and seeds: 1 to 2 grams per serving

All, including almonds, sesame seeds, Brazil nuts, black walnuts, peanuts, sunflower seeds, filberts, pecans, and pumpkin seeds

---

FIBER FACTS

How much fiber is enough? Currently women are eating about 12 grams of dietary fiber a day, and men 18 grams. The cancer-prevention recommendation is 20 to 30 grams, or 1 gram per 100 calories. Interestingly, therapeutic diets for diabetes may prescribe as much as 70 grams a day, while our Paleolithic ancestors consumed well over 100 grams a day. But the optimum amount is still a subject of debate.

On the flip side, there's little or no fiber in meat, cheese, eggs, and milk; butter, margarine, oils, and sauces like mayonnaise and salad dressing; fruit and vegetable juices; honey, soft drinks, sugar, white flour, most processed foods, and alcohol. Unfortunately these raw materials comprise the majority of our in-house menus—and certainly the bulk of our restaurant options.

In the absence of fiber-filled Cinderella foods, the ugly stepsisters, fat and sugar, elbow their way in. And they're so calorie-rich they're spoiled rotten.

In the following examples, foods on the left side of each equation match those on the right in number of calories.

3 beers or Cokes and a 7½-ounce bag potato chips	=	6 apples and 1 loaf whole wheat bread
8 ounces rib roast	=	10 ears corn on the cob
10 ounces sirloin steak	=	5 baked potatoes
1 cheeseburger	=	18 cups air-popped popcorn
1 strawberry milkshake	=	8½ cups fresh strawberries
1 slice cherry pie and ½ cup vanilla ice cream	=	117 fresh sweet cherries

There are lots of folks who can put away three beers and a bag of chips, or a milkshake, or a plain cheeseburger. But the high-fiber calorie equivalents on the right sound more like an all-you-can-eat Guinness world's record.

Even so, there's no need to give up all your favorite dishes just because they are on the low-fiber list. Simply cut your portion size, then add extras to boost the total fiber of your meal or snack. Try these suggestions:

- Love huevos rancheros? Add fresh tomato, onion, and bell pepper, serve with corn tortillas and salsa, and finish off with fresh pineapple or papaya.
- Cheese soup your weakness? Combine with crisp bran crackers, a crunchy salad, and an apple for dessert.

- Enjoy chicken or pork—just less of them—with stir-fried Oriental vegetables and brown rice.
- German sausage could benefit from side dishes like new potatoes in jackets or hot yogurt-potato salad, lightly steamed cabbage and apples, and dark sourdough rye.

Like the "What's wrong with this picture?" puzzles, at first glance this cafeteria menu appears fairly balanced and nutritious. However, it's suffering from a serious fiber deficiency. Can you come up with nutritious substitutes to fix the no-fiber problem?

> Apple juice
> Cheerios and milk
> Eggs
> Toast and butter
>
> Grilled cheese sandwich
> Onion rings and pickle slice
> Tomato soup
> Saltines
>
> Roast beef and gravy
> Rice
> Spinach
> Roll and butter
> Vanilla wafers
> Milk

Now see what Living Lean suggests:

~~Apple juice~~	Fresh apple
~~Cheerios~~ and milk	Nutri-Grain flakes
~~Eggs~~	Whole wheat French toast with
~~Toast and butter~~	slivered almonds
~~Grilled cheese sandwich~~	Grilled tofu sandwich on pumpernickel rye
~~Onion rings and pickle slice~~	Garden salad with sunflower seeds
~~Tomato soup~~	Chunky vegetable soup
~~Saltines~~	Whole grain flat bread
Roast beef and gravy	
~~Rice~~	Spicy red beans
~~Spinach~~	Brown rice
Roll and butter	
~~Vanilla wafers~~	Oat bran muffin
~~Milk~~	Fresh peach

SHOPPING WITH FIBER IN MIND

We went on a free shopping spree (no purchases) at the largest natural foods grocery and the best-stocked supermarket in our area, looking for fiber in all the right places. This is what we turned up:

- Fresh produce—you can't go wrong here.
- Dried beans and peas—they're all good, so make a point to try 'em all.
- Breads—darker, heavier breads including pumpernickel rye and 100 percent whole wheat are best bets, but for fussy families, a lighter granola-type bread would be a good transition. Also sample just-for-fun novelties like whole wheat breadsticks, pizza crust, and burger buns.
- Crackers—same cautions as for bread. Also check ingredient listing for salt and fat. Whole wheat matzos, Swedish rye, rye crispbread, whole grain flatbread, puffed brown rice cakes, and brown rice crackers are low in fat—and tasty.
- Cereals—Shredded Wheat, Grape Nuts, and old-fashioned oatmeal are still among the best whole grain, sugar-free choices. Try also Nutri-Grain with or without raisins, Nutri-Grain Nuggets, oat bran flakes, and hot cereals like oat bran, Ralston, and Roman Meal.

For some foods, only the nutrition department at the supermarket matched the variety at the natural foods store:

- Cereals—if you (or the kids) like Cheerios, Cream of Wheat, and Rice Krispies, you'll love the whole grain versions, marketed under a variety of brand names. We also found plain *whole* grain puffed cereal, including millet and wheat, and granola with less fat and sugar. You have to be a label detective in this area.
- Grains and pasta—meal-makers like millet, whole wheat noodles, and vege-burger mixes are often sold in bulk so you can try a little before you buy a lot.
- Quick mixes—who said whole grains take too long? If you find yourself in constant jeopardy of assault by a deadly cupcake, try some alternatives: whole grain bread, muffin, and cake mixes (you add the fresh bananas, carrots, and apples), whole wheat gingerbread, buckwheat pancakes, oatmeal cookies, and whole grain corn bread are all eat-em-up treats. Hot out of the oven, none of them will linger long on your kitchen counter.
- Bran—you can create your own bran-enriched breakfast by sprinkling one or two teaspoons of wheat or oat bran over your whole grain cereal. Or add it to stew, soup, vegetable juice, meat loaf, casseroles, stuffing, breading, or baked goods. Too much wheat bran can cause bloating or trigger allergy in some people; oat bran usually has no side effects. Start slowly with either, and make sure to include a variety of high-fiber foods—not just bran—in your eating plan.

🥫 LABEL LINGO

The label isn't lying when it says "made from unbleached wheat flour" or "enriched flour or cornmeal." What it forgets to tell you is both of these are stripped, white, fiberless starches, often with a little whole grain flour, bran, or caramel thrown in for color.

Ignore the waving wheat fields and earthy colors on the front, and head straight for the fine-print facts listed under ingredients. Whole wheat or another whole grain should be listed first; and unless it specifies "100 percent whole grain," it probably isn't.

"You mean I can have popcorn?" "Wow—I *love* pasta." "I could eat fresh peaches every day." For Living Lean students who have shunned carbohydrates for years (or guzzled them in guilt, regardless), high-fiber eating is nothing but good news. Like a kid in a carbo store, you can pick among dozens of choices and have lots of fun cooking—and eating—new, creative combinations. But start slow and simple, and build up your repertoire gradually. The easiest way to stock fiber foods in your pantry is to make simple changes in your shopping list. How about one nutritious switch each week?

Instead of these . . .	Try these
elbow macaroni	whole wheat ribbon noodles
orange juice	orange
soda crackers	Swedish rye crackers
popsicle	frozen pureed fruit
tomato juice	fresh tomato
candy bar	raisins
sweet roll	whole grain English muffin or bagel
frozen waffle	buckwheat pancakes
potato chips	almonds
pretzels	popcorn
white bread	whole wheat bread
doughnut	bran muffin
puffed rice	Shredded Wheat
onion dip	bean dip
white rice	brown rice
butter cookies	oatmeal cookies
hamburger	vege-burger

GRAIN AND BEAN CUISINE

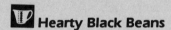 **Hearty Black Beans**

Vary the flavor of these basic beans by adding a can of tomato sauce or a chopped jalapeno pepper; or vary the beans. For kidney beans, omit the powdered spices and add a few shakes of red pepper sauce.

2 cups black beans	1 teaspoon oregano
8 cups water	1 teaspoon cumin
1 onion, chopped	1/2 teaspoon dry mustard
2 cloves garlic, pressed	1/4 teaspoon salt (or to taste)
1 bay leaf	

Simmer all ingredients covered for about two hours, or until beans are very tender.

1 cup = 2 Grain/Starch, 1 Protein

Pineapple Oat Bran Muffins

You can use crushed pineapple instead of chunks in these muffins, but the latter retain more flavor during cooking. Freeze a batch of muffins and serve hot for a tasty, filling snack.

1 1/4 cups canned, unsweetened pineapple chunks, well drained
   (cut each chunk in half)
2 cups oat bran
1/2 cup whole wheat flour
1 tablespoon baking powder

1 tablespoon fresh grated orange peel
1/4–1/2 teaspoon salt
3/4 cup skim or low-fat milk or buttermilk
2 eggs
1/3–1/2 cup honey or maple syrup
2 tablespoons vegetable oil

Combine dry and wet ingredients separately, and mix well. Add liquids to dry ingredients, and stir just until moistened. Spoon into 12 lightly oiled muffin tins or foil liners. Bake at 400 degrees for 12 to 15 minutes.

1 muffin = 1 Grain/Starch, 1 Fat

LEAN BEAN COOKERY

Learn to cook one kind of bean, and you can cook 'em all. Bring to a boil one cup dried beans and recommended amount of water. Lower heat and simmer, covered, until very tender (improves digestibility). To shorten cooking time, you can presoak one cup beans in three cups water overnight. Season with onion, garlic, chili powder, cilantro, parsley, bay leaf, cumin, ginger, mustard, tomato, or any herbs, but add salt—if used— just before serving (it toughens beans and increases cooking time). Bean appetit!

Bean Variety (1 cup)	Water (cups)	Cooking Time (hours)
Adzuki	2	1 1/2
Black	3	2
Black-eyed peas	2	3/4–1
Kidney	2 1/2	1 1/2
Lima	3 1/2	1 1/2–2
Lentils	2	1/2–3/4
Navy	2 1/2	2–2 1/2
Pinto	2	1 1/2–2
Red	3	2–2 1/2
Split peas	3	1–1 1/2

✓ PRACTICE: FOCUS ON FIBER

Post the list of Outstanding Fiber Foods in your kitchen and select your meals and snacks from it as much as possible during the coming week. You might also want to include one or both of these suggestions on your Practice Diary:

- Eat more whole grains—at least two servings every day this week.
- Eat more dried beans, peas, and lentils—one serving at least three times this week.

Dried beans are easy to locate, but searching out authentic whole grains may require some sleuthing. Refer to the Shopping with Fiber in Mind guidelines and the grocery list substitutions. If fiber is all new to your diet, try to use a variety of whole grains like oats, barley, or brown rice instead of just wheat and wheat bran products—they take a little longer to get used to.

Tame Your Appetite

It happened yesterday, it already happened today, and it will no doubt happen again tomorrow: you got hungry. Even though it happens *every* day, you still forgot to stuff your pockets with fruit, or to make a sandwich for lunch when you left home this morning. A breakfast pastry and coffee obligingly shuts down stomach grumbling for a while, but by one o'clock the pangs are ordering "Eat something or *die*." All that's in sight—or smell—is the crispy chicken shack, the pretzel palace, the deli dog, the quick-dip ice cream cart, and the trusty vending machine. You feel compelled to gorge but settle for a hot dog instead.

Never a stranger, though, Hunger is back again—double strength this time— by four o'clock, and no wonder. Thus far, the most intense part of your day has been fueled by a sugar-coated roll, a hot dog, and two "diet" sodas. You're still short 65 percent of your daily calorie quota.

Five-thirty finds you desperately ransacking the ice box. The verdict: nothing quick and nutritious, so the candy bar hidden in the freezer will have to do. "I'll just diet tonight," you decide righteously while crumpling the wrapper. But your body has other ideas. By the time dinner is on the table, you're overhungry. The unfed animal appetite orders "Eat, eat" and you obey, gobbling too much, too fast, hardly able to taste or enjoy the food going down the hatch. You never intended to finish the day in this ravenous condition. How did it happen?

SET THE TIMING: GRAZE, DON'T GORGE

If you're hungry all the time, or overhungry at the wrong times, your timing may be off. The obvious antidote for hunger is to eat—and eat often. The best way to do this is to add between-meal snacks while cutting the size of main meals. In other words, graze, don't gorge. Think in terms of six small, equal-spaced meals instead of one or two big ones. Living Lean students who adopt this schedule rarely complain about being hungry—that is, unless they graze on all the wrong things.

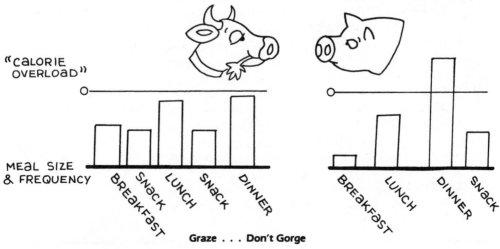

Graze . . . Don't Gorge

"But eating during the day makes me feel sluggish." Maybe you're eating too much at a sitting—and then sitting some more. You're an even better candidate for between-meal snacks; they help sustain your energy and allow you to feel satisfied with smaller meals. Also make sure your lunch includes a protein source. Too much carbohydrate, and you're likely to feel drowsy instead of energized afterward.

Take a look at your Eating Diary once more. Do you see clusters and holes in your eating routine? If so, distribute the same number of calories more evenly. For this college student, 6½ hours between lunch and dinner and 14½ hours between "bigger snack" and lunch are too long to go without eating:

Breakfast	none
Lunch	1:00 P.M.
Dinner	7:30 P.M.
Big Snack	9:00 P.M.
Bigger Snack	10:30 P.M.

"But we've always been told not to eat until we're hungry." If you skip (or skimp on) perfectly good meals, you're likely to get hungry later when there's nothing nutritious for miles around. As you tumble into bed tonight, resolve to try a new tack tomorrow: plan to get hungry (because you will eventually), and then eat before you do.

If you are weak-kneed at 10:00 A.M. and 4:30 P.M. every day, plan a snack at 9:30 A.M. and 4:00 P.M. If you always come home from work and ravage the refrigerator before starting dinner, eat a muffin or drink a carton of milk while you're waiting for the commuter train. Set up a consistent eating schedule and your hunger clock will stop going off when you aren't prepared for it. If Living Lean testimonials are any indication, your reward for simply carrying an apple in your briefcase or toting sunflower seeds in your pocket or purse may be well worth your effort. For one thing, more snacks could mean fewer total calories.

HUNGER BUSTERS

- Eat breakfast, or a more *substantial* breakfast, with a little protein or fat, especially if you're plagued with afternoon hungries.
- Eat a snack or meal every three or four hours during the day; it doesn't have to be much—sometimes a bite or two will do.
- Eat a real snack, while sitting down, *before* you start dinner or while it's cooking; try to keep your paws off the dinner foods until dinner, when you can be conscious of what and how much you're eating.
- Eat something before you go—whether it's a cross-country drive, a late dinner out, a beer and chips party, or a long meeting with only coffee for refreshment.
- Take something with you when you go to the movie, the beach, or the park; otherwise, the concession will probably snatch your small change.
- Keep a list of good and easy snack ideas handy, and add a few of them to your grocery list each week.
- Some of the most popular snacks can provoke hunger rather than satisfy it; take it especially easy on the Spoilers—sugar, salt, caffeine, and alcohol.
- Eat mostly fiber foods, say Living Lean students, and you won't have to deal with going hungry at all.

EAT OFTEN (AND YOU'LL EAT LESS)

How do you make a fat rat? You tell him the kitchen is closed until dinnertime so he can't nibble all day and spoil his appetite. After a week of frustration, he learns to eat a lot of rat chow (5 to 15 percent more) at his one big meal, and he ends up gaining 30 percent more fat weight as a result. This could be bad news for those of the human species who alternately stuff and starve themselves because they don't have time (or so they say) to eat on a regular schedule. A different study found rats deprived of food all but one hour a day are more likely to choose sugar water than nutritious rat chow when they do eat. If this translates to soda pop instead of bagels for overhungry people, skipping meals and snacks could do double damage.

If you're a confirmed member of Overeaters Unanimous, set the Timing now for Quantity (and perhaps Quality) Control. Though it sounds crazy at first, you will not only be less hungry, you will probably eat less (and store less surplus body fat) if you eat more often—every three to four hours if possible. In other words, if you graze, you'll be less likely to gorge. Just choose *what* you graze on carefully.

On the other hand, there are a few people, like Rhonda, who really need to batten down the cupboards. Rhonda's one-day Eating Diary had 40 entries. Each time she would pass out peanut butter graham crackers or fruit juice popsicles to one of her three preschoolers, she'd have a bite, too, often with a cheese and Frito chaser. There was nothing that looked like a real breakfast or lunch anywhere on her diary, and not a veggie in sight.

And that's the main problem with quick foods and no prepared meals: the vegetables—especially cooked veggies—seem to disappear. If you have unlimited access to food during the day, designate a definite time for meals, and schedule a reasonable number of fillers in between them. If you have to, leave a note on the fridge that says, "Safe Deposit Box: Only open for snacks at 10, 2, and 4."

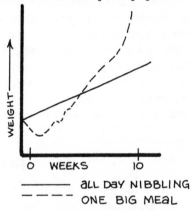

Meal Frequency and Weight Gain in Growing Rats

SNAPPY SNACKS

Whoever told you to avoid snacking was way off target. Post this list on the back of a kitchen cupboard door and go for good snacks. When you try a new idea, check it off; then add your own inventions to the list.

- Fresh pear with Neufchatel or "light" cream cheese
- Half hard-cooked egg with bran crackers; low-sodium tomato juice with no-salt seasoning or a dash of hot pepper sauce
- Unsweetened applesauce with cinnamon and nuts or a spoonful of granola
- Whole wheat blueberry muffin with a cup of skim milk
- Frozen yogurt: stir 1 cup plain, low-fat yogurt into a cup of commercial fruit yogurt and freeze
- Toasted, unsalted soybeans
- Tart or sweet lemonade: juice of ½ lemon, 1 cup sparkling water, 1 teaspoon honey or to taste

- Plain yogurt mixed with a spoonful of frozen orange juice concentrate, topped with fresh orange slices
- Blender gazpacho: 1 cup tomato juice, ½ stalk celery, ½ green onion, ¼ to ½ cucumber, 1 to 2 teaspoons lime juice, sprinkle of garlic, few drops of hot pepper sauce
- Fresh peach with low-fat cottage cheese and graham cracker
- Trail mix: salt-free sunflower or pumpkin seeds, almonds, raisins, dried apricots
- Main-dish leftovers or soup with a salad and a cup of low-fat milk
- Fruit juice soda: mix equal parts cranberry-apple juice, orange juice, or another fruit juice with plain carbonated water (Nature's answer to soft drinks)
- Carob cocoa: heat 1 cup low-fat milk, 1 to 1½ tablespoons carob powder, ½ teaspoon vanilla, pinch of cinnamon, 1 teaspoon honey or to taste
- Fresh apple with part-skim mozzarella cheese
- Club soda with grapefruit juice; a handful of granola
- Tomato-buttermilk cocktail: combine ½ cup tomato juice, ½ cup buttermilk, and a dash of no-salt herb seasoning
- Summer punch: 1 cup orange juice, ⅓ cup pineapple juice (unsweetened), 1 tablespoon fresh lime juice, 1 cup plain carbonated water, ice cubes
- Hot chicken stock or broth, fat-free; whole wheat low-salt pretzels
- Plain low-fat yogurt with a handful of fresh blueberries; raisin–oat bran muffin
- Whole grain rye crackers with part-skim mozzarella cheese
- Frozen grapes, frozen banana slices (dipped in lemon juice before freezing)
- Raw veggies—carrot sticks, celery sticks, cucumber chips, cherry tomatoes— and powdered dip mix prepared with plain low-fat yogurt and blended cottage cheese in place of sour cream
- Popcorn Parmesan: sprinkle 1 to 2 tablespoons grated Parmesan cheese over air-popped popcorn
- Apple tea: combine equal parts apple juice and herbal tea, such as peppermint; serve iced with lemon
- Peanut butter spread thin over brown rice cakes, topped with raisins
- Potato crisps: slice raw or lightly steamed new potatoes into ¼-inch rounds; bake at 350 degrees for 15 to 20 minutes (or until crisp and golden), turning once

SNACK-ATTACK SOLUTIONS

A little extra effort in planning your snacks can help prevent hit-and-run nutrition. Replace regular chips and sodas with better choices, for example, and you've scored a major improvement.

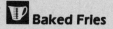 **Baked Fries**

Bake potatoes in a 400-degree oven for 15 minutes. Spray a cookie sheet with nonstick spray. Cut potatoes into ¾-inch sticks and arrange on cookie sheet. Bake at 400 degrees for 25 to 30 minutes or until golden.

8–10 fries (1 small potato) = 1 Grain/Starch

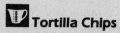 **Tortilla Chips**

Stack three corn tortillas; fold and break, or cut, into six triangles. Bake on a cookie sheet at 325 degrees for 5 to 10 minutes or until crisp but not brown. Or allow to dry in a warm oven until crisp. Store in airtight container.

6 chips = 1 Grain/Starch

Spicy Guacamole

1/2 cup mashed avocado
6 tablespoons plain low-fat yogurt
1 tablespoon fine-chopped red
  onion
2 teaspoons lime juice
1/4 teaspoon garlic powder
1/4 teaspoon dark chili powder
pinch salt

Combine all ingredients.

3 tablespoons = 1 Fat

Spinach Dip

1 10-ounce package frozen
  chopped spinach
1 cup low-fat cottage cheese
1/4 teaspoon garlic powder
1/4 to 1/2 teaspoon soy sauce

Thaw and drain spinach. Puree all
ingredients in a blender until
smooth.

1/2 cup = 1/2 Protein, 1 Vegetable

✓ PRACTICE: FILL IN THE SNACK GAPS

This is your week to eat more—specifically, more often—so enjoy yourself. If you have one of those watches that beeps, set it for half-past breakfast and again at half-past lunch—the optimum times to reach for a nutritious snack. Plan to get hungry, then eat *before* you do.

Consult the list of Snappy Snacks if you're fresh out of easy ideas for nutritious fillers. Log one or two of the Hunger Buster techniques on your Practice Diary, too, if you like. Then use them whenever the opportunity arises. If the whole concept of snacking is alien to your lifestyle, remind yourself that a few extra snack calories now could save lots of extra binge calories later. Eat more often.

The Caffeine Scene

Lela said she'd give it a try. Cold turkey—no caffeine—for ten days, just to see if she felt any different without it. Giving up regular coffee would be a snap, she said. After all, she normally drank only one cup a day, first thing in the morning. Two days later, she was on the phone, incredulous at her misery. "My head feels like it's being sledgehammered ever since yesterday morning, and I'm so tired I can barely function. I can't believe it! It's like I'm going through withdrawal from some addictive drug."

Not everyone suffers upon saying "so long" to caffeine. But a few unlucky souls get depressed, disoriented, nauseated, constipated, and quite irritable. Despite such blatant evidence, caffeine still seems like a bosom buddy. It offers a reliable lift when you're down, whether bleary-eyed at the jangle of the alarm clock or fagged-out before the five o'clock rush.

But caffeine is more fiend than friend, insidiously sapping your energy so that it can—like the dope-pusher—pick you back up again, taking all the credit and none of the blame. A revealing study compared the effect of caffeine (equal to 1 1/2 and 3 cups of coffee) on habitual users and abstainers. Noncoffee-drinkers felt normal with a placebo, but were jittery and nervous and complained of upset stomach with the real thing. Coffee-lovers, on the other hand, experienced sleepiness and irritability when given a placebo, but felt alert, contented, and less irritable with genuine caffeine.

Caffeine is a true stimulant, increasing your heart rate, triggering irregular heartbeats, making you breathe faster, and stepping up the release of stress hormones. Only 250 milligrams of caffeine during the day—about 2 to 3 cups of coffee—can hike blood pressure as much as 10 points. The elevation is transient, but for many people caffeine intake is as regular as the morning sun and significantly more frequent. Caffeine also increases the secretion of stomach acid, making it one of the few definite no-nos for ulcer patients. Then there's caffeine's diuretic effect—annoying at least and dangerous at worst—washing a number of important nutrients out of the body, including calcium and other electrolyte minerals. But the verdict is still out on other health risks, including a link to birth defects, fibrocystic breast lumps, and increased mortality from heart disease.

For calorie-watchers, tea, coffee, and artificially sweetened sodas have always appeared on the "unlimited" food lists. But your body needs and wants food, not caffeine—especially in the morning, when consumed calories are put to good use. A typical breakfast of coffee and toast or juice puts a temporary hold on your appetite, but it will resurface with a vengeance later in the day, as many Living Lean students can attest. (Skip the morning caffeine and watch as your mid-afternoon munchies mellow out by the end of the week.) Caffeine does increase metabolic rate by as much as 10 percent, but sly side effects like tension, nervousness, and fatigue may lead the "dieter" directly to the refrigerator. If your goal is to become lean as well as healthy, then you need caffeine like a fish needs a bicycle.

This table shows the caffeine extremes in popular drinks and over-the-counter drugs.

CAFFEINE COUNTER

Sources of Caffeine	Caffeine (mg)
Hot coffee, 5-ounce mug (drip)	115*
(perc)	80
Instant	65
Decaf	3
Hot tea, 5 ounce mug	40
Imported, black tea	60
Instant	30
Iced tea, 12 ounces	70
Cola beverage, 12 ounces	40–60**
Chocolate milk or cocoa, 6 ounces	5
Chocolate, 1 ounce	20
Fast-relief pain medication	60
Cold tablets and pain medication	30

*Strong coffee will have more caffeine.

**Of the soft drinks, sugar-free Mr. Pibb and Mountain Dew have more caffeine; Dr. Pepper, Pepsi, and RC Cola have less.

It's understandable if you are reluctant to give up your caffeine companion, even temporarily. Parting with caffeine may seem more painful than the end of a sweet summer romance—at first. But if you value your independence, it's best to say goodbye to an unhealthy relationship. Those who have successfully kicked the habit never regret it.

Of course, life may not be quite as fast or stimulating sans caffeine; then again, it may offer unexpected rewards. Instead of waking up to smell the coffee every day, perhaps you'll find yourself stopping to smell the roses.

☑ PRACTICE: TAPER OFF MR. CAFFEINE

Are you ready to take the "America's cup" challenge? Go cold turkey on caffeine for one week, just to see if you feel any different without it. People who are especially sensitive to the chemical might want to extend this practice a second week to completely eliminate any possible withdrawal fatigue. If the thought of Living Lean without caffeine makes you tremble like the caffeine shakes, try some of these tips for tapering off:

- Pour a whole cup of coffee, but drink only half.
- Percolate or steep your coffee or tea for less time.
- Avoid strong or black tea or dilute with water, ice cubes, or fruit juice.
- Switch to instant coffee (less caffeine) or coffee blended with roasted grains.
- Use caffeine-free soft drinks.
- Experiment with caffeine-weaning: the first week, mix part decaf with part real coffee (or other caffeinated beverage); the second week, combine equal parts "fake" and real or use a "50 percent less caffeine" coffee; the third week, make it mostly decaf; and the fourth week, you're home free (caffeine-free, that is).
- Sample true alternatives like 100 percent grain "coffee," herbal tea without caffeine, carob drinks, carbonated water, fruit juice, milk, or plain water.
- If you constantly feel in need of a pick-up, investigate the Quality Control of your eating.
- For relaxation and tranquility, try aerobic activity, rest breaks, deep breathing, or a brisk shower.

✐☑ Practice Diary Two

"Okay, I'm ready to lose this fat now." Great—Living Lean is behind you 100 percent. Just keep in mind there is a productive change sequence, outlined first in the Introduction, that will help you achieve your goal.

- **Fitness first.** If you didn't begin walking or working out last week (Week One), get going now on your major muscle and metabolism makeover. Although fitness walking is a "no experience necessary" occupation, if you're a true novice, read ahead to Chapter 3 for some practical pointers.
- **Identify the problem.** Now that you know how, when, and where your appetite leads you astray (as reported in your Eating Diary Analysis this week), make some simple changes that will make a difference.
- **Quality and Quantity Control.** By eating more foods with fiber—and by eating more often—you can earn more nutrition while spending fewer calories.
- **Fitness again.** Though you might not be aware of it, your good eating and aerobic efforts will begin to play important roles in burning up calories and regulating your appetite by next week (Week Three). It takes a month or more to enjoy *visible* results, but remind yourself that the valuable changes in your metabolism and body composition already under way will make it easier for you to stay lean once you become lean.

If these techniques seem too elementary or if you are impatient to *see* the changes in your body composition, you can adopt the calculated eating approach described in Chapters 4 and 6. However, you may not need it. As many Living Lean participants have discovered, *it is possible to lose fat without deliberate calorie restriction*, so long as you (1) increase aerobic activity above your present level and (2) make wise food selections, primarily those high in fiber (and low in fat).

RECORD MEALS AND SNACKS

SUNDAY

MONDAY

TUESDAY

WEDNESDAY

THURSDAY

FRIDAY

SATURDAY

PRACTICE DIARY TWO

Practices	Day							Notes
	Su	M	Tu	W	Th	F	Sa	
Continue Fitness Walking								
Focus on Fiber								
2–5 servings whole grains per day								
3 servings cooked dried beans per week								
Fill in the Snack Gaps—morning/afternoon								
Taper Off Mr. Caffeine								

✓ = yes, I did try;   ✓✓ = yes, I did well!

Suggested Practices

- Complete the Eating Diary Analysis and note problem areas to work on.
- Read the Label Lingo to find a new brand of bread, cereal, crackers, or pasta that is authentically whole grain.
- Shopping with Fiber in Mind: make one nutritious switch in your grocery list each week, exchanging a low-fiber food for a high-fiber food.
- Tame Your Appetite: try to eat your meals and snacks at approximately the same time each day.
- If you snack all day instead of eating meals, plan at least two seated meals daily.
- Record your meals and snacks one or more days this week in the space provided here.

WEEK THREE

Earn an "F" for Fabulous Fitness
   *One Look Back, Full Speed Ahead
Aerobic Engineering: Move It to Lose It
   Aerobic Alternatives
   *Be Heart Smart
   Comfort Equals Safety
Living Fitness
   *How Fit Are You? A Fitness Walking Test
   Fitness Logistics
   *Walk It Off
   Food as Fuel
   *Practice: Aerobicize Your Schedule
Salt: Shake It Easy
   *Salt of the Earth
   Spice It Right
   Practice: Skimp on Salt
   Practice: Refocus on Fiber
*Practice Diary Three

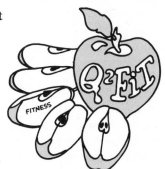

Earn an "F" for Fabulous Fitness

Thinking about skipping the exercise stuff in this book? Stop right there! This chapter is *really* important.

Just ask Bobbie. She watched her husband go from a lean jogger to a hefty nonjogger (after a leg injury) in less time than it takes to moan, "I'm bored." "I couldn't see where he altered his food intake at all," puzzled Bobbie, "but the fat has piled on just the same."

Or ask Hazel. Six weeks of castle steps, shopping sprees, and tortuous scenic overlooks successfully sheared the inches that had resisted every "diet" known to man—in spite of enough food to ransom a queen. "I would never have believed it!" she exclaimed upon checking her new measurements.

No doubt you have heard aerobic activities are good for you, but do you know how good? Enough to earn an "F" in the Success Formula for Living Lean. We're talking Big Benefits here: let us count the ways.

First, aerobic activity expands your lung capacity, which helps carry oxygen and nutrients to your brain and every cell in your body, while removing carbon dioxide and other wastes. Thus, you can think and work with more energy and endurance and less fatigue. Are your hands and feet always cold? Aerobic activity improves your circulation. At the same time, it strengthens and tones all your muscles, including the master muscle—your heart. Though you may never have to run for your life or save a drowning person, at least you will be physically in shape to do so.

Just a few additional bonuses you can look forward to by being fit: lower blood pressure and a slower heart rate, which means your heart has to work less. Your blood won't clot so easily, and blood fats like cholesterol and triglycerides decline, reducing their tendency to build up in your artery walls. Meanwhile, the HDL or "good guy" of cholesterol increases. In other words, more physical fitness means less heart disease. It also means less colon cancer and, for women, less reproductive cancer and osteoporosis as well. Recent evidence indicates fit people not only live better, they live longer, too.

Such lifetime benefits might entice you up off the sofa once or twice. But what keeps people perpetually in motion—hiking, biking, or shooting baskets—are the more immediate physical and psychological rewards. Mad at the boss? Depressed? Tense? No self-confidence? Physical activity can improve all of the above, according to various research studies. One group of women who participated in a walking and jogging program reported they felt better, enjoyed social functions more, and were less—not more—fatigued at the end of each day. Are you one of those people who carts a barrel full of complaints to your physician, ranging from stress headaches, insomnia, or premenstrual syndrome to indigestion or constipation? A little aerobic activity may be just what the doctor should order.

The benefits could be even more rewarding. For instance, you could take the backpacking trip you wouldn't have dared before. You might climb the pyramid with the rest of the tour group, instead of again saying, "I'll just wait at the snack bar." You would enjoy square dancing without all the huffing and puffing. You could play volleyball with the gang at the family reunion. And with less worry and more productive action, you might earn a pat on the back rather than a stern lecture at your next medical checkup. Best of all, your daily aerobic break offers a chance to escape from the office and its pressures or the house and its drudgery for a half hour or more each day. Not a bad return on a minimal investment.

"Fine, fine. But what does fitness do for fat?" Obviously it burns calories. But perhaps more important, it builds muscle, increases metabolism, and enhances the burning of fat for fuel. Though you can't make fat cells disappear, aerobic activity siphons more storage fat out of the cells than "dieting" does.

Walking or jogging also offers a diversion from TV game shows and tempting snacks in the refrigerator. At the same time, it decreases at least one hormone (insulin) that can trigger terminal munchies. Last, it enhances a positive mood, reduces stress, and heightens appreciation for rather than disapproval of your body. As one student aptly put it, "It not only makes me feel good, it makes me feel good about myself."

CLEAN-AIR CONTRACT

If you're a smoker, the single most important thing you can do for your health is kick the habit. But you probably know that already. If you can quit for 24 hours, you're well on your way; six months, and you've got it licked. An occasional cigarette after that doesn't mean your attempt has failed, either. Try toothpaste, breath spray, mouthwash, mints, or sugarless gum after dinner instead of lighting up. Since the craving only lasts 5 or 10 minutes, distract yourself with a brisk walk or deep breathing—anything to focus your attention elsewhere.

Friends told Charlie he couldn't quit his three-pack-a-day habit after 30 years; they told him he'd get fat; they told him he was too nervous to quit. There was no end to what they told Charlie, and he got sick of it. So he quit smoking all by himself, without consulting anyone. And to further prove them wrong, he did not add any extra fat-pounds because he walked after meals, he cut way back on meat, alcohol, and television (all cigarette cues), and he ate more fruits and vegetables. He even started drinking milk.

Most people gain no more than 8 to 12 pounds when they quit smoking, due to a slowing of metabolism. Aerobic activity can prevent a lot of that metabolic decline. Regardless, two lungs are priceless when compared with a few extra pounds. (And you'll save your skin from premature aging, too.) The Q^2FiT Formula can help you with this project, so add Stop Smoking to your Practice Diary if you'd like. You couldn't give yourself a more fantastic gift.

 ## ONE LOOK BACK, FULL SPEED AHEAD

Look back a moment to your years as a kid. Were you active? How about as a teenager? Was there any change in your activity when you left home? Attended college or started working? Quit a job or left school? Got married or had children? Moved to another town or neighborhood? Bought the VCR or joined an exercise club? Injured your back or retired? Gave up recreational activity or took up a new sport? Ask yourself why for any "yes" answer, and then "What can I do about it?"

Now pinpoint significant changes in your body composition—good or bad— and jot down when they occurred and, if possible, why. Did a change in activity precede an increase in body fat?

Change in Body Composition	When	Why

Most important, can you think of some immediate and lasting benefits that will encourage you to become an "active citizen"? List as many as you can think of here.

Immediate benefits:

Lasting benefits:

Aerobic Engineering: Move It to Lose It

To be totally fit, you can pursue activities that make you stronger (to lift that single suitcase aboard your international flight), faster (to chase down the last bus home), more flexible (to fold yourself, yoga-style, into a subcompact car), more agile (to keep up with a four-year-old at the playground), and provide endurance (so you can hit every store at the shopping mall). Only sustained activities provide what you need most, however: whole-body fat-burning and aerobic heart-and-lung conditioning.

Activities that accomplish this are as close as the nearest fitness class. People who would never routinely climb on a bike or jump in a pool are easily lured into a gym after work to sweat and sing along with Billy Joel or Dolly Parton. With a quality videotaped program, you can burn calories in the comfort and privacy of your own living room, at any hour of the day or night.

Don't overlook the rewards a group has to offer, however. You will make new friends, and in a semicrowded class you will also discover there is no such thing as an average body, much less an ideal one. Instead, you see infinite variety in size and shape—from gazelles to gorillas. (It is interesting that gazelles can be awkward and clumsy while gorillas can be delicately graceful, and both can become aerobically fit.) When you unconditionally accept everyone else's shape and fitness level in a relaxed sociable setting, it helps you accept your own luck-of-the-draw as well. If you are intimidated by muscle-and-fashion-show aerobics, keep hunting until you find a program that allows for, and encourages, individuality. Somewhere there is a class that is exactly right for you.

NO STRAIN, NO PAIN

"Keep going—twenty-five, twenty-six—make it burn!" barks the exercise drill sergeant. But according to Jacki Sorensen, whose aerobic programs are among the oldest and safest, overworked muscles are especially vulnerable to fatigue, cramping, and injury. To enjoy the fitness gain without the muscle strain, shop carefully before you pay your fee.

- An aerobics class should be fun and challenging, never boring, and music is a must—the Lamaze method of physical conditioning.
- Quality aerobics shoes and a wood floor or other resilient surface help prevent common impact injuries, as do routines without repetitive movements.
- Calisthenics like leg lifts, which concentrate on certain body parts, will tone the muscle under the fat but will not reduce the fat over the

muscle; whole-body aerobics are best for decreasing body fat, and 30 to 45 nonstop minutes are a recommended minimum.

- Your pulse should climb neither too high (above 75 to 85 percent of your maximum heart rate) during routines nor fall too low between routines.
- A low-impact or low-level class is probably most productive for initially out-of-shape and overfat folks.
- An aerobics class should meet two to three times a week but never more than four; hiking, biking, and swimming can round out your fitness week.

AEROBIC ALTERNATIVES

Dr. Kenneth Cooper of the Aerobic Center in Dallas has his own ranking of the best all-around aerobic sports, and cross-country skiing heads up the list. Though definitely seasonal, it burns an awesome number of calories. Between seasons you might investigate sports equipment that simulates cross-country skiing. For this demanding sport, it pays to get in shape ahead of time.

Then there's swimming, rated second, but often the first step for those who are truly underfit and overfat. It allows a whole-body workout without the danger of overheating (a significant problem for fat-insulated people), and those with injuries or arthritis can move in most any direction with water serving as a protective cushion. Underwater even heavyweight landlubbers are light as a feather, and the feeling is pleasantly addicting. Once you see how swimming tones and firms your chest and shoulders (which get little help from the sports ranked third, fourth, and fifth), you may have to be coaxed out of the water rather than into it.

Running is the third best aerobic choice, but it will always be number one in the hearts and soles of dedicated runners. Running—or even its less aggressive cousin, jogging—is a good option for busy people; you can accomplish a lot of aerobic calorie-burning with a minimal time investment. Occasional joggers quickly find themselves addicted to the peace, the pace, and the power of running, and find it's fairly easy to stick to it.

When you get tired of the same old sights, simply vary the route. In fact, you can run away to just about anywhere in the world with only your passport and running shoes for companions. And if you need extra incentive now and then, you can find it in a competitive runners' club or a free-spirited run-for-fun event.

⚓ SWIM AND TRIM

Here are some suggestions to help you get in the swim—and stay there.

- Protect your coiffure with a shower cap, then grab a kickboard and splash your calories away. If you need them, get a snorkel for breathing, a wet suit for warmth, or goggles to guard against chlorine.
- Even a flounderer will burn calories, but don't hesitate to sign up for a swimming skills class—it's fun.

- When you get tired of traditional swim strokes, try aqua exercises (offered at YMCAs and fitness clubs). In chest-deep water, you can jog or do continuous calisthenics like bobbing and stretching.
- Another idea: strap on a pair of fins, hook your toes over a rope, and swim in place; or grab the rope and practice your kick; or simply tread water.
- If you are always overhungry and overtired after a swim, slow your conditioning heart rate 10 beats and cut back to a 20-minute swim.

Bicycling is another great nonimpact sport, so it ranks fourth on the list. True aerobic cycling in downtown Manhattan may kill you before it conditions you (wear a helmet, please), but an indoor stationary bicycle offers all-weather access plus safety and privacy. Even though you can read, watch TV, or recite the Bill of Rights at the same time, some find it a little too dull to pedal and pedal without ever going anywhere.

Out on the streets you may have to put in a bit more time, though—say a ride of 45 minutes to an hour—to get the same fat-burning advantage of a half-hour jog. (That's because you spend some of your time coasting.) On a stationary bike, however, the tension knob allows you to select the intensity of the ride and thereby pedal away your calories faster.

PEDAL PUSHING

If you are shopping for a stationary bike, try it out for comfort at least 10 minutes straight before you sign on the dotted line. Many people find a recumbent model more comfortable, but whatever your choice, be prepared to spend $200 plus for a really good one. Always adjust the seat properly: when the pedal is nearest the floor, your foot should be flat and parallel to the floor, with your leg almost fully extended.

Besides offering a gentle alternative to the pounding of jogging, biking is fun and an efficient means of transportation. With a bike rack on your car, you can take aerobic fitness with you—from a ride through the Great Smoky Mountains National Park to a tour down the California coastline.

The key to most of these aerobic sports, though, is an excess of initiative, plus recreational togs to start, and then a shower to finish. That's why the sport ranked number five is also the number one all-around lean-builder and fat-burner: walking.

The first time you did it, Mom and Dad squealed with delight and took your picture. And you've been doing it ever since, because walking is a natural. Most anyone can walk—anytime, anywhere—sans special equipment outside of a sturdy pair of walking shoes. You can sneak off for a walk when you need it most, without telltale perspiration and gym shorts to give you away. And whether your goal is getting lean or just getting from here to there, you'll find aerobic walking is easy to weave into your daily routine. It's also simple to pick up again after a layoff—another reason walking is *the* most popular recreational activity.

Walking is a sociable sport; you can have a heart-to-heart conversation right in the middle of a workout. Plus it's one of the few aerobic activities men and women with varying fitness levels can do together. Create a rendezvous time and place for neighborhood walkers, and you'll rarely walk alone. If you're feeling a bit contemplative, on the other hand, walking by yourself allows you to enjoy rare solitude.

It's easier to control the intensity of a walk than a run, which helps you stay within your aerobic limit and avoid injuries. Walking also allows you to maintain your workout longer without getting out of breath or pooping out; and a long, slow calorie-burn is the optimum way to dig into body fat stores. Three miles an hour, or 20 minutes per mile, is a good pace for long walks—the U.S. Army ought to know! But as you get in better shape, pick up your feet and the tempo. If it still feels too tame, try race-walking to add some spice to the sport. True to its label, you can fan the competitive flame and burn major-league calories without the physical impact and joint stress of jogging.

Like runners, Living Lean walkers tend to get hooked. If you become a walker for life, you're in good company—with the likes of Johnny Appleseed, who wandered for 40 years; William Wordsworth, who logged 14 walking miles each day; and Thomas Jefferson, who said, "Of all exercises—walking is the best."

But what if your sole goal is to metabolize body fat? Is walking worth the effort? You better believe it is. During a landmark year-and-a-half study, one group of women walkers shed an average of 22 (and as many as 38) scale-pounds—without cutting back on food at all. In fact, most of the women claimed to be eating more. After years of losing and regaining the same pounds, they found they could maintain or increase these results simply by adjusting their time spent walking.

A study by Drs. Peter Wood and Abby King of Stanford suggests fitness even beats out dieting. Participants who were instructed in "diet" techniques lost 16 scale-pounds, while those given exercise instruction without any mention of food restriction lost only 10. A three-year follow-up found the "dieters" right back where they had started, however, while the original exercise group had regained little of their lost fat. Results like these could put us nutritionists right out of business! Interestingly, the "dieters" lost a pound of lean for each 4 pounds of fat, while the exercisers kept their lean; the lean loss might have been responsible for their rebound (see Chapter 5). Regardless of rationale, the outcome was unequivocal: *Don't fudge on fitness!*

⚉ GET FIT ON FOOT

There are ways to get more of a walking workout with the same number of miles logged:

- Walk faster (the easiest way).
- Swing your arms vigorously or pump them, with elbows bent—you'll burn 5 to 10 percent more calories (much more effective than hand weights, which can throw you off balance).
- Walk or hike uphill, and give your thighs and buttocks a thorough workout; plus you'll burn twice as many calories on a 10-degree slope as on the flatlands—even more on a really steep incline.
- Walk downhill; after every up comes a down, but you continue to burn more calories because you are braking.
- Walk (carefully) over an uneven surface, like a dirt trail, a soft sandy beach, or a dry creek bed.
- Instead of tiny mincing steps (as if you were still clipping around in uncomfortable dress shoes), try a longer stride, pushing off with your toes.

- Try walking backward to warm up and cool down—it will stretch the opposite muscles and take stress off your knee joints.
- Forward or backward, walk tall and proud with your tail tucked under to strengthen flabby abdominal muscles.

BE HEART SMART

When you say "aerobics," people invariably picture themselves sweating up a storm or gasping for breath. The truth is, your metabolism is aerobic even while you're reading this book—though it would take years of aerobic couch-sitting to burn off unwanted fat and you would never condition your heart and lungs that way.

On the other hand, many so-called aerobics classes may actually be *anaerobic* (without oxygen, or too high-intensity) for you. When you can't easily catch your breath, you are approaching your aerobic limit. Exceed it, and your body must switch to glucose-predominant fuel while fat-burning metabolism comes to a screeching halt. Lactic acid starts to build up, and exhaustion may set in. People who are overfat, out of shape, or who have noninsulin-requiring diabetes may bump into this aerobic limit at a lower workout intensity than normal people.

Primary Fuel	Metabolism	Heart Rate
Glucose/glycogen	Anaerobic (very high intensity, exceeding the aerobic limit)	Greater than 75%* or 85%** stress level— the aerobic limit
Body fat	Aerobic (optimum heart and lung conditioning and fat-burning)	60%* or 70%** stress level
	Aerobic (very low intensity)	Less than 60%* or 70%** stress level

*Suggested level for all overfat people as well as those of below average or low fitness, based on the Fitness Walking Test in this chapter. (People with health problems should get an individualized recommendation.)
**Suggested level for lean, active people and for those of average or better fitness.

So that you don't exceed your aerobic limit, make sure you can comfortably breathe and simultaneously carry on a conversation while you are working out. Or monitor your heart rate as follows:

- First, locate your pulse on the side of your neck (below your ear, just under your jawbone).
- Second, determine your heart rate per minute while you are sitting and resting; count the number of beats in 6 seconds (count the first beat at zero, not after a second has passed), then add a zero to the total. For instance, if you count 13 beats in 6 seconds, your heart rate is 130 beats per minute.

Your resting heart rate: _____

- Now, using the guidelines in the chart above, determine your conditioning heart rate zone:

220 – your age = your maximum heart rate: _____

your maximum heart rate × .60 or .70 (60% or 70% stress level) = your optimum conditioning heart rate: _____

your maximum heart rate × .75 or .85 (75% or 85% stress level) = your aerobic limit and your maximum conditioning heart rate: _____

your conditioning heart rate zone: _____ to _____
  optimum   maximum

If you stay within your conditioning zone, you can be confident that your heart and lungs are getting a productive workout and you are disposing of body fat at the same time.

At first, check your heart rate often—before you set out, after several minutes of brisk walking, at the halfway point, and at the end of your jaunt. Five minutes after the end of your workout, do a recovery heart rate check. It should be less than 120 (or less than 100 if you're over 50). If it's not, you overdid it! As you become fit as a fiddle, your resting heart rate may slow down, saving your heart thousands of beats every day and adding years to your heart-life-expectancy.

COMFORT EQUALS SAFETY

Strained muscles. Shinsplints. So stiff and sore you can't move the next day. It doesn't have to be that way! Practice commonsense prevention, and warm up a few minutes before heading out—a slow walk, a gentle swim, a leisurely bike ride. After your muscles are warm, they can better stretch without overstretching. Do each one of the following stretches gently, without bouncing, and hold for 20 to 30 seconds. Breathe deeply throughout, relaxing into the stretch, without tensing other muscles. In other words, don't hold your breath or tighten up. Yanking on a muscle till it hurts won't help it, but it could injure it.

If you are short on time, the calf stretch is probably your best choice, especially if you hobble around in high heels all day. Use a wall or a tree for support if you need to. Just remember to keep your upper body perpendicular to the ground, your back straight, and both heels on the ground. Repeat with both right and left calves.

Now, grab your left thigh from behind with both hands and gently bring it toward your chest. You can also do this stretch lying on your back on the floor. Repeat with your right thigh.

Simple Stretches

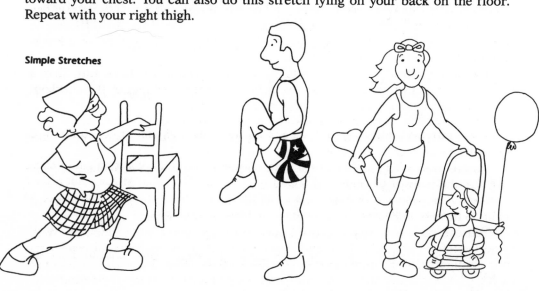

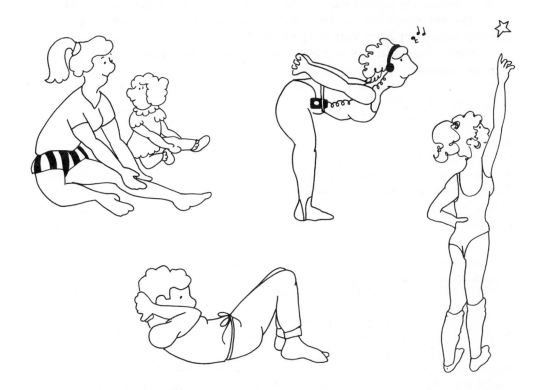

Reach behind you, grabbing your right ankle or shin. Bring it gently toward your rear end, keeping your knee pointed down if possible, and hold. Repeat with your left ankle.

To stretch your hamstring (back-of-thigh muscle), sit with your left leg extended in front of you, with your right leg bent so the sole of your right foot rests against or close to the inside of your left leg. Lean forward from your hips, keeping your head and chin up, and hold. Then repeat with your right leg.

Last, stand tall and clasp your hands behind you. Gently lift them, feeling the stretch in your shoulders. Hold, relax, and repeat. If you are quite flexible, you can do the same stretch while bending at the waist, as pictured. If you are inflexible or stiff, you can sit in a chair and lean forward so that your chest rests on your knees and your head and arms droop, relaxed, toward the floor.

By the way, these are great stretches whenever you feel tight or stiff. Take a real stretch break from paperwork every hour. Rotate tired feet in the checkout line. Give shoulders a lift and a shrug during a long drive.

Here are a few more stretches if you have time.

Stand tall, knees relaxed, and reach for a star with your right hand. Hold until you feel a good stretch, then repeat with your left hand.

Rotate your shoulders in a circle to the front, as if you were pedaling a bicycle with them. Now reverse and pedal backward.

Gently and slowly nod your head forward, then roll to the right, then forward again, to the left, and forward once more, in a semicircle. Repeat.

You can do a new and improved curl-up to strengthen your abdomen. With knees bent, feet flat on the floor, and fingertips cradling the back of your head, curl your shoulders and the upper part of your back off the floor. To get the most out of each curl, breathe out and push your lower back against the floor, tightening your abdomen. Concentrate on using your abdominal strength, not your shoulders or back, to lift you off the floor. As a variation—and to help you keep your lower back planted on the floor—scoot right up next to a chair. Lie on your back, but rest your legs on the seat of the chair. Do 10 to 15 curls.

When you get to the end of your workout, don't stop suddenly. Instead, walk, bike, or swim slowly to prevent blood from getting temporarily trapped in your arms and legs, shortchanging vital organs. Stretch again thoroughly, this time to prevent morning-after stiffness (it really works).

A typical aerobic hour (or 45 minutes) could look like this:

- 5-minute warm-up
- 5-minute stretch
- 30 to 45 minutes of fun aerobics
- 5-minute cool-down and stretch

If aerobic activity feels good, you'll be more likely to pursue it without prompting. Since nothing beats happy feet, start from the bottom with the basics: at least one pair of comfortable shoes designed expressly for sport walking or jogging. Another savvy idea—all-function shoes that brag style, yet offer enough traction for a brisk walk to the bus stop.

Develop a wardrobe that not only looks good but facilitates movement as well, so you don't feel compelled to change clothes every time an opportunity for action presents itself. If you find yourself more physical in a warmup suit than a three-piece suit, start acquiring a classy collection of sports togs.

Since safety is synonymous with comfort, take it from the top: a hat will reflect the sun's wicked rays in summer and conserve body heat in winter. Select fitness apparel that allows you to perspire, yet keeps you from getting chilled. In cool weather, choreograph your hike so the wind is at your back on the final stretch. On a hot or humid day—or even a cool, dry one—drink a couple of glasses of water 30 to 15 minutes before you set out. (Better to make a pit stop behind an obliging bush than to feel symptoms of heat exhaustion coming on with nary a water fountain in sight.) Take a canteen along on an extended trek, and then be sure to drink more water after you get back to camp. You can see that water is the key. When it's too hot out, head for a cool pool or an air-conditioned gym. You may need a little salt (from foods, not salt tablets) during the first steamy days of the year, but your body should adapt to a normal sodium requirement after a week or two.

If your heart rate is low on a given day but you feel fatigued, don't push for speed; you can always walk a little longer should you decide to. If your heart rate is unusually high, even though you feel like a million, drop back. Once the adrenalin is flowing in a noisy aerobics class or a handball tournament, you may not notice the pain, or the fact that you're exceeding the fat-burning speed limit. Better to err on the side of safety.

Don't ignore warning signs! If your pulse is erratic or way too fast, you suddenly feel chilled on a hot day, you experience chest pain or nausea, or you feel dizzy, overheated, or uncoordinated, stop and sit or lie down. Elevate your feet if possible. Seek medical assistance as soon as you're able.

There are other indisputable signals that you've overdone it: extreme fatigue two hours after a workout, an exhausted feeling that lasts beyond a day, a recovery or resting heart rate that's too high, chronic anemia, or aches, pains, and injuries. Sleeplessness and more than an occasional charley horse may also be a sign of too much of a good thing (which becomes a bad thing). Gently but firmly stretch a cramped calf or foot, lightly massaging the muscle and breathing deeply at the same time. If the muscle is quite sore or definitely injured, ice is the preferred treatment. Chronic insomnia and muscle cramps sometimes respond to increased fluid intake or may indicate a need for more dietary calcium or magnesium, especially in women. If the problem is that you are consistently overexerting, the obvious solution is to cut back and spare yourself a lot of unnecessary aspirin and x-rays. Remember:

- Eat before you get too hungry.
- Drink before you get too thirsty.
- Rest before you get too tired.

FUN WITH FITNESS

Can you smile in the midst of your workout, or is your attitude more befitting the Grim Reaper than winged Mercury? Is physical activity a relief from stress or one more stress added to the daily jumble? Do you enjoy the moment or are you preoccupied with pouncing on the scale when you get through? If you think competitive thoughts like "go faster," stress hormones are released, which can raise blood pressure, cause water retention, decrease immunity, and increase blood cholesterol—hardly health-promoting fitness goals!

Another problem: the adrenalin high from all-out effort may be counterproductive when it comes to burning fat. As you slam the ball into outer space, your body must hand you a glucose energy fix to fuel your shot while fat-burning is shut down, at least momentarily. Thus sprint-and-stop sports like tennis or high-intensity fitness classes may not deliver the fat reduction you desire if you fail to work or play at a consistent aerobic level. Even if you're a walker, it doesn't pay to push your pace to the absolute limit.

In short, take your fitness project seriously, but not *too* seriously. And if your personality is as hard-driving as your backhand, explore the mellow pleasures of some sustained, mid-level aerobics every now and then.

Living Fitness

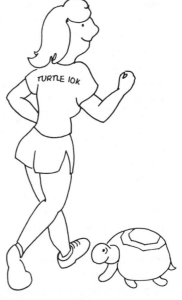

It's no crime to be out of shape—you've got lots of company. But it's foolish to pretend you're in shape if you're not, and play a hard game of volleyball, shovel a foot of wet snow, or haul a deer carcass halfway down a mountain, only to end up putting yourself out of commission. Not to mention that the pain could discourage you from making more constructive fitness resolutions.

So start from where you are now—slowly—because you've got plenty of time. The pace can be simultaneously comfortable and productive; in the race against body fat buildup, the tortoise wins, not the hare. Actually, winning the race is less important than crossing your self-set finish lines every day. And as your fitness improves, you'll discover your speed, stamina, even your aspirations, will accelerate all by themselves.

Slow and Steady Is the Way to Go!

✏ HOW FIT ARE YOU? A FITNESS WALKING TEST

A small hill looks and feels like Mount Everest. A couple of flights of stairs and you have to halt and catch your breath. You don't need a fitness test to tell you you're out of shape. Instead, start with only 5- or 10-minute walks several times a day, and give yourself plenty of time to work up to a mile. *Then* you can take this test.

To take the Rockport Fitness Walking Test:

1. Walk slowly 5 or 10 minutes to warm up, and stretch a bit.
2. Now walk as fast as you comfortably can, covering one mile around a measured track at a school or stadium. (One Living Lean student had her husband cheer her on from the grandstand while he clocked her with a stopwatch.)
3. Note how long it takes to complete the mile, and check your heart rate immediately upon finishing. (For this check, count your heartbeats for 15 seconds and multiply by 4.)

Time: _____   Heart rate: _____

4. Compare your results with the fitness standards in Appendix B. You might want to adopt the progressive walking program outlined for your fitness level. Or you might prefer to walk whenever and however far you please, just for the fun of it.

Fitness level: _____

FITNESS LOGISTICS

If the Fitness Walking Test confirms that your current physical endeavors consist solely of chasing rainbows, climbing the corporate ladder, or jumping to conclusions, then now is the time to outline your get-fit strategy. Once you have decided which aerobic option appeals to you and where you can do it, the next question is . . .

When? Some folks use an aerobic jaunt to rev up before a busy day; others prefer to aerobically unwind after all the chaos has subsided. Try both, one week at a time, and see which feels better and works into your lifestyle. (Ozone and other pollutants rise after dawn, peak around noon, and then fall after the evening rush hour. If you live in a smog-choked area, it might be a good idea to avoid outdoor aerobics during peak pollution times.)

Research currently favors the early-bird workout for better fat-burning. One study found that three-quarters of calories burned before breakfast were fat while only half of those burned before supper were fat. But total calories burned were a bit higher in the late afternoon, so take your pick. Also, overfat folks burn the most calories when they work out before a major meal; that's good because strenuous activities on a full stomach could place a strain on your heart or jostle your food right up.

Best idea: an energetic swim or walk first thing in the morning or before the evening meal; a leisurely digest-your-dinner, walk-the-dog stroll while the supper dishes soak. A family of eight traditionally parades through our neighborhood each night, complete with baby buggy and assorted-sized kids bouncing balls and tossing Frisbees. Take your cue from an English proverb that says, "After dinner sit awhile, after supper walk a mile."

How often? You can't store fitness, so your feet should hit the dusty trail on a near-daily basis. Research shows that four to five outings a week are significantly better for fat-burning than three outings a week. "That schedule doesn't work for me," announced one restaurant manager. "It's too easy for two days off to stretch into a week down the drain. I have to plan to walk every day, then really try to do it. That way it's more like a routine." He has a point.

Once- or twice-a-week sports like aerobic classes, tennis, volleyball, or golf offer fun and fitness but little fat-burning unless you fill in the aerobic gaps. The most dramatic fat-loss stories are told by students who really work at logging the miles, as you might have guessed. Biking, swimming, and walking are so safe you can enjoy them daily as long as you recover enough energy to do them every day. On the other hand, impact sports and max-out exertion require scheduled off or easy days or an occasional low-stress activity to allow you to recuperate.

If you slack off too long, though, your problems are reversed: after a month or two of doing nothing, you can say goodbye to most of the benefits you worked so hard to accrue. Like an insurance policy that has lapsed, you have to start all over. "I ran track in high school," provides a great collection of mementos for the scrapbook but not a lick toward lasting fitness. So go for it: four days a week is a productive minimum, but even one day a week is better than none. *The minimum is four, but try for five.*

How long? The key here is to count the minutes, not the miles. Look at your watch, strike out on your walk-'n-jog, and don't stop until you've clocked at least 30 minutes. This magic number is a minimum for promoting effective fat loss, according to a number of studies. But if time is precious, a 10-minute walk every day adds up to 60 hours (and 24,000 calories) of walking in a year—an easy way to ward off 7 sneaky pounds of fat. Only got five? Then take five! Consider it a victory walk if you get out from behind your desk at all. Don't get trapped in the all-or-nothing rut.

Should you find yourself with time heavy on your hands, however, milling and munching about the house or office, there's no reason not to work up to a longer trek. Beyond 30 minutes of effort, proportionately more fat is burned as fuel, as the following chart illustrates. On the weekend, make it more play and less workout. Pack up the family for a long bike ride or hike at the state park, and your aerobic hours will positively sail by. *From 30 to 45 minutes—and that's a minimum.*

How fast? If you love living in the fast lane, you may have to downshift to reach the optimum cruising speed for fat-burning metabolism—your conditioning heart rate zone. When you exceed your aerobic limit, you burn glucose calories in preference to fat calories. You also burn *out* faster at full throttle, which means fewer total calories burned. High-speed, high-intensity effort can overstress bones, joints, and muscles, and it has a strange and mostly unfavorable effect on appetite (Chapter 5). If you have a choice, *don't go faster, go longer.*

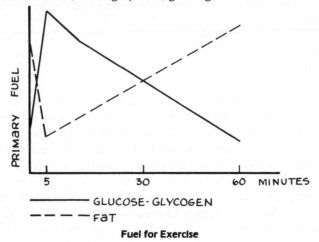

GLUCOSE·GLYCOGEN
FAT

Fuel for Exercise

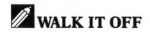

WALK IT OFF

How fast do you walk? If you don't have a measured track to check your walking speed, count the number of steps you take in 10 seconds. Then use this chart to find your speed.

Average Female	Average Male	Walking Speed
20–21	16–17	3 miles per hour
24–25	18–19	3 ½ miles per hour
27–28	20–21	4 miles per hour

Your walking speed: _____ miles per hour

60 minutes + _____ miles per hour = _____ minutes per mile

CALORIES BURNED IN A HALF HOUR OF WALKING

Miles Per Hour	Minutes Per Mile	Weight in Pounds					
		100	120	140	160	180	200
3	20	90	110	130	150	170	190
3½	17	110	130	150	170	190	210
4	15	125	150	175	200	225	250
4½	13	140	170	200	230	260	290
5	12	160	190	225	265	305	345

Based on your walking speed and body weight, determine how many calories you burn in 30 minutes. Multiply by 1.5 to find calories burned in 45 minutes or by 2 to find calories burned in 60 minutes.

Calories burned per day while walking: 30 minutes _____ 45 minutes _____ 60 minutes _____

Calories burned per day: _____ × _____ walking days per week = _____ calories burned per week

Last, determine how many pounds of fat you will dispose of each week with the above schedule.

Calories burned per week: _____ ÷ 3,500 calories (equals 1 pound fat loss) = _____ fat-pounds burned per week

Note: As a result of Quality Control eating and beneficial changes in metabolism and appetite, Living Lean students often see body fat disappear faster than predicted, and research supports their observation.

FOOD AS FUEL

If you've always thought of food as something to fill you up when you're hungry, it's time to start thinking like a budding athlete. Food is fuel, and carbohydrates are your key to peak performance. They are the sole fuel for high-intensity speed sports and a primer fuel for moderate, drawn-out activities like hiking, biking, and everyday chores. But don't run out and buy a year's supply of jelly beans and soda pop. Simple sugars are useful only when you are in the middle of an extended run or hike. If you stoke up before you set out, sugar shuts down mobilization of your own body fuel—including fat fuel—and often triggers a rebound crash in your blood sugar.

Instead, it's nutritious carbos you're after: complex starches like whole grain bread, cereal, and pasta, potatoes and other starchy vegetables, plus fruits for natural sugars. These fuel-efficient carbos keep your body engine running long and lean. But hold the grease that is usually drizzled *over* your carbohydrates. Too much cheese, butter, rich pastry, or fried food is like water in the gas tank.

A little body protein is broken down during every vigorous workout and then rebuilt—sometimes augmented—in between. If you do enough and then rest enough, you will build muscle. (Thus a little more *rest* might help the overexerciser grow lean.) Studies indicate protein needs are slightly increased for the athlete in training (that's you). But Americans already eat more protein than their bodies know what to do with. Just make sure you don't skimp on calories ("dieters" take heed), so that food protein can be used primarily for body building and repair, not for energy needs.

FUEL-EFFICIENT CARBOS

You rarely run out of glycogen since your body keeps about a day's worth stocked in your liver and muscles. But when it's running low, complex carbohydrates are the best foods to restock it.

What if you accidentally eat more carbos than you need to replace missing glycogen? The overflow is more easily burned for energy than stored as fat, since it costs extra calories to make body fat from carbohydrate. In other words, carbohydrates may be less fattening than other food calories. (When animals overeat carbohydrates one day, they eat less food the next day; this appetite adjustment does *not* occur when they eat too much fat.)

It seems only logical to try to burn more body fat (aerobic fuel) than body glycogen (anaerobic fuel) during your workout. And since burned-up body fat may be harder to replace when you eat carbohydrates, that's exactly what you *should* eat. Keep your body machine running lean with fuel-efficient carbos. *Burn fat—eat carbos.*

Even with the proper fuel mix to propel you down the highway—high in carbohydrate, moderate in protein, and low in fat—body fat still won't burn spontaneously. It's a complicated biochemical process requiring dozens of enzymes assisted by vitamin- and mineral-containing helpers called coenzymes. Here's the impressive starting lineup:

- B vitamins, particularly thiamin, are key players in generating aerobic energy. A major shortage means less endurance, early exhaustion, and a depression of the aerobic limit.
- Vitamin B_6 is needed to stimulate growth hormone, which in turn triggers the breakdown of body fat for fuel.
- Aerobic means "with oxygen," so iron—the oxygen carrier in your blood—is a critical team member, especially for women.
- Calcium and zinc help delay the onset of muscle fatigue.
- Electrolytes like sodium, potassium, calcium, and magnesium keep fluids in balance and maintain proper muscle contraction.

And there are even more participants. Aerobic metabolism is a true team effort, and you can't win if you're short one of these players. Thus, calorie and nutrient deficits from chronic "dieting" could throw the fat-burning game if you're not careful. On the other hand, an extra player on the field is just wasted; repeated studies show that nutritional supplements won't squeeze a better performance out of an adequately nourished person.

The time-tested strategy will always be your winning strategy—the Success Formula for Living Lean. And to avoid pointless penalties, save most of the low-nutrient sweets, fats, and alcohol for your victory celebration.

FOR FLEET ATHLETES

If you have trained regularly for a couple of years but still have body fat to burn, examine your aerobic fuel. Is it high-octane, premium calories or watered-down regular? Sure, you get to eat more when you do more, but exactly what are you eating, and how *much* is more?

If you are a high-miler, keep in mind your body more resembles a well-tuned sports car than a chugging '52 Chevy. You get more miles per calorie than your sedentary friends, which is okay as long as you keep putting in the miles. If you have to cut back on distance, do so gradually, or you may discover a few extra pounds on your luggage rack until your body adapts.

Think twice before pushing toward an "ideal" percentage of body fat, too, even though your goal is to maximize performance. If you must resort to unnatural acts—near starvation or 70 miles of running a week—to achieve it, you are most likely pursuing someone else's body blueprint, not your own, and your performance may actually suffer.

PRACTICE: AEROBICIZE YOUR SCHEDULE

To make fitness fit in, schedule your aerobic intentions as if they were really important appointments (they are!), and then plan around them. Don't let anyone or anything nudge you out of your convictions or off your schedule, because only you will have to reap the consequences—good or bad. You'll find surprisingly more energy and more time to complete more tasks if you're physically fit. You're not wasting time—you're gaining it.

A Typical Aerobic Week

Here's the plan. Create a schedule that not only announces what you're going to do but also when, where, and for how long.

S	M	T	W	T	F	S

Days per week:

Minutes per day:

Primary aerobic activities (days per week/minutes per day):

Busy-day activities:

Bad-weather activities:

Current fitness level:

Fitness level in four months (goal/actual):

Fitness level in one year (goal/actual):

Special fitness goals:

Salt: Shake It Easy

If you like card tricks, you might appreciate this challenge. Pick out the four saltiest foods in this list: a bowl of corn flakes, a small bag of potato chips, a slice of Sara Lee Dutch Apple pie, an ounce of salted peanuts, half a cup of Jell-O Instant Chocolate Pudding, a small serving of salted french fries from McDonald's, a McDonald's chocolate milkshake, and four saltine crackers.

The hand is quicker than the eye if you selected crackers, nuts, chips, and fries. They contain 109, 123, 133, and 165 milligrams of sodium, respectively. By comparison, the corn flakes contain 260 milligrams, the shake 300 milligrams, the pudding 460, and the pie 585, courtesy of food-processing magic. If you're not wise to such hocus-pocus, the numbers can go even higher—and visible salt or a salty taste are not always reliable indicators.

SALTY DECEIVERS

These are some salty foods* that might fool you:

1 cup Total cereal	375 mg
3 ounces Chicken of the Sea tuna	400
3 Aunt Jemima pancakes	643
1 packet Quaker instant oatmeal	280
1/2 cup Minute Rice Long Grain and Wild Rice	570
10 ounces Campbell's Chicken Noodle soup	1,200
3/4 cup Kraft macaroni and cheese	845
6 ounces Campbell's V-8 juice	555
McDonald's cheeseburger	767
2 slices Pizza Hut Thin and Crispy Supreme Pizza	1,200
Weight Watchers Turkey Tetrazzini	1,443
1 cup Chef Boy-ar-dee Beef Chili with Beans	1,005
1 1/2 ounces Lite-Line Sharp Cheddar Flavor Slices	668
Arby's roast beef sandwich	880
Burger King Whopper	990

*Product ingredients change constantly; the only way to stay sodium-wise is to read labels.

One small teaspoon of salt is worth over 2 grams (2,000 milligrams) of sodium. Since we are supposed to eat only 1 to 3 grams of sodium per day, it's easy to see why so many people get too much. Currently, women are within the acceptable range for sodium intake if they don't add salt at the table or while cooking. Men, however, eat too much sodium—3,600 milligrams' worth—even before sprinkling salt over their food. In fact, 75 percent of all the sodium we eat comes hidden in processed foods.

People who are more than 40 years old, black, or prone to high blood pressure are more likely to be salt-sensitive and to experience a hike in blood pressure when they eat salt. But everyone else should shake it easy, too. Although salt has no calories, it does tend to cause water retention. Since excess water is excess weight, a wild (and salty) party weekend can tilt the scale with misdirected guilt come Monday morning. A salt overload could also be hazardous to your disposition. Laboratory rats fed too much salt appear edgy and unable to deal with new situations—in other words, stressed out.

Salt generally hangs out with an unwholesome crowd. Not only do sugar and fat calories sneak in on salty coattails, there's a more insidious problem. Eating sodium causes your body to lose potassium, and a lack of potassium has been implicated as one culprit in both hypertension and water retention. When you eat highly processed foods, for example, you not only *get* less potassium, you probably *lose* more because of the excess sodium.

In this showdown between processed and unprocessed foods, you can see that where sodium is, potassium isn't:

Processed Foods	Sodium (mg)	Potassium (mg)
1 cup tomato bisque soup	872	263
2 ounces extra lean lunch-meat ham	810	198
½ cup canned green beans	200	82
1 slice apple pie	476	100
Unprocessed Foods		
1 tomato	10	255
2 ounces sliced roast pork	54	317
½ cup fresh green beans	4	373
1 apple	1	244

Even slightly processed foods like frozen peas have more sodium (70 milligrams) than fresh peas (4 milligrams); canned peas are even saltier (186 milligrams). If you stick to plain, unadulterated foods, you will come out ahead—or, more appropriately, behind—in your sodium intake.

SALT OF THE EARTH

One or two salty foods won't be a problem for you unless you're on a sodium-restricted diet. But too many choices from this list could add up to a salty snag in your efforts at Living Lean.

Circle the foods below you eat often, then try to cut down on the least nutritious of them first.

Beverages: softened water, some public water supplies, sugar-free soft drinks, some mineral water

Quick breads: waffles, pancakes, biscuits, cornbread, muffins, crackers, pastry, cake, pie (fried or homemade), boxed cereals, some quick-cooking cereals

Vegetables: almost any canned vegetable (except low-sodium), including canned tomatoes, tomato juice, tomato paste, green beans, peas, lima beans, corn, asparagus, beans and franks, sauerkraut

Snacks: salted or buttered popcorn, pretzels, potato chips, corn chips, tortilla chips, salted nuts, olives, pickles, snack dips

Processed meats: bacon, hot dogs, cured ham, sausage, cold cuts like salami and bologna, smoked meats, corned beef, dried chipped beef, beef jerky, salt pork

Canned meats and packaged dinners: tuna, anchovies, herring, lox, chili, stew, ravioli, macaroni and cheese, canned or packaged soup

Dairy foods: processed cheese—spreads, American cheese, "diet" cheese, most others; natural cheese—Cheddar, cottage cheese, most others; commercial pudding, cocoa mix

Fast foods: pizza, cheeseburgers, hamburgers, breaded frozen fish, salted french fries, most fast foods

Frozen foods: dinners, "light" entrees, pot pies

Condiments: soy sauce, bouillon, broth, marinade, gravy mix, cooking wine, mustard, steak sauce, barbecue sauce, chili sauce, ketchup, reduced-calorie mayonnaise and salad dressing, regular salad dressing, salted margarine and butter, nondairy creamer, meat tenderizer, MSG, lemon pepper, onion salt, garlic salt

Medicines and additives: Alka Seltzer gold, sodium propionate, sodium saccharin, sodium bicarbonate (baking soda), monosodium glutamate, baking powder

SPICE IT RIGHT

One woman who abruptly omitted all salt from a fairly nutritious diet found herself eating mounds of greasy, fatty snack foods as a result. Even though her blood pressure remained quite normal, her figure did not. She decided her snacks were a disguised excuse to replace the missing salt, so she added a little salt again in cooking, and sure enough, the unwanted junk foods faded out of the picture. As they say, whatever works!

Here are a few suggestions for slacking off on salt:

In Cooking

- Omit or cut down on the amount of salt in the recipe, then let each person add salt or seasoning to taste.
- Recipes for vegetables, pasta, and cooked rice or cereal often call for salt, but it's all right to leave it out.
- You can more easily get by with just a tad of salt than none at all, say experienced chefs. Judicious amounts of salty condiments like mustard, horseradish, Tabasco sauce, taco sauce, ketchup, pickles, olives, barbecue or steak sauce, salad dressing, marinade, or even reduced-sodium soy sauce add more flavor than would plain salt.
- Replace garlic salt, onion salt, lemon pepper, bouillon, and commercial broth with salt-free or reduced-sodium alternatives.
- Cook with wine (but not super-salty cooking wine or sherry) for a fancier flavor; use lemon and fresh pineapple to tenderize meat. Worcestershire sauce is fairly low in sodium.
- Try not to season in black and white (just pepper and salt); colorize with dozens of different herbs, and be daring in your combinations: a pinch of red pepper or curry on fruit, cinnamon on cheese, mint in milk, lemon juice on baked potato.

At the Table

- Try herb blends and salt substitutes for sodium-free seasoning; if you have health problems, check with your physician before buying a high-potassium salt substitute—some people should not use it. If you are simply trying to cut down on a hefty salt habit, powdered sea kelp or "lite" salt could be a first step; both contain sodium, but good amounts of potassium. Except for a few trace minerals, sea salt is identical to regular salt.
- Make salt more of a bother; leave it in the cupboard or use a shaker with only two or three holes.

In Food Choices

- Yeast breads (bagels, rolls) have less sodium than quick breads (biscuits, muffins) unless you use low-sodium baking soda and powder in cooking.
- When shopping, look for the brand with less sodium, like low-sodium tomato juice or salt-free crackers; then add a bit of your own seasoning. Even if you use salt as your seasoning, it will probably be less than the food manufacturer would use.
- Fast foods, most restaurant foods, and Oriental foods are usually higher in sodium, so complement them with unsalty fruits or vegetables.

SPICE UP YOUR LIFE—WITHOUT SALT

You've tried one or two herbs, but you haven't tried them all! For good flavor without salt, experiment with basil, black pepper, coriander, cumin, chili powder, dill, celery seed, curry, marjoram, oregano, onion, garlic, or tarragon. Lemon, herbed vinegar, tomato sauce, parsley, and bell pepper will also add zest to plain foods.

✓ PRACTICE: SKIMP ON SALT

You *can* shake the salt habit. According to one study, it takes no longer than four to six weeks (and probably less time for most people) to make a fairly permanent low-salt impression on your taste buds. If you don't like plain unsalted chips or can't eat your popcorn or eggs unless they are coated with salt, now's the time to try cutting down. Just for this week:

- Stash the salt shaker somewhere away from the table.
- Try not to salt during cooking, but do season generously with herbs and spices.
- Compare brands to find the one with the least sodium; add your own seasoning to salt-free brands.
- Make a point to skirt two or three foods from the Salt of the Earth list this week; note them on your Practice Diary.
- Be aware that processed foods, many restaurant foods, and most fast foods will have four times more sodium than a similar dish prepared at home.
- If you can't follow all the above suggestions, just choose one idea for this week and record it on your Practice Diary.

☑ PRACTICE: REFOCUS ON FIBER

Week Two may be gone for good, but the focus on fiber is far from forgotten. In fact, the fiber practice is so valuable it bears repeating. If you enjoyed eating oat bran cereal, whole grain pasta, and pinto bean dip last week, do the same—just more of it—this week. If you're already sold on beans and grains, then take the pledge for fresh (or frozen) fruits and veggies, too.

- Whole grains—at least three servings daily
- Dried beans, peas, and lentils—one serving at least four times this week
- Fruit—at least two servings daily
- Vegetables—at least three servings daily

Keep up the good eating and before you know it, you'll be a permanent member of the fiber fan club. Better yet, join now—the benefits are terrific.

🖋☑ Practice Diary Three

For 95 percent of us (and that probably includes you), aerobic activity is the Missing Link to living a lean life and the single most important thing you can do for your health (after you quit smoking). In fact, evidence indicates inactivity is as bad for your health as having high blood pressure or cholesterol or smoking a pack of cigarettes a day.

Wouldn't it be nice to thumb your nose at the next "miracle diet," rip out all the other chapters in this book, and never have to worry about wardrobe stretching again? Glance once more at the Big Benefits listed at the beginning of this chapter. Wouldn't it be nice to have a few of them for your very own? With moderate aerobic activity you can be confident that bona fide fat is being dismantled, not some other body part you'd just as soon keep!

Since it took years to acquire your extra fat, it's only fair to allow enough time to properly and aerobically dispose of it. What's important is not your fat quotient in six weeks but rather in six months or six years. And will you be healthier as a result of any changes?

Unfortunately, patience is not an attribute of most "professional dieters," the medical establishment, or our culture in general, so you may have to get assertive—with your family, your friends, the magazine predictions, and, most important, yourself. In fact, your fitness investment is much like a retirement savings account, with one striking difference: you not only reap the ultimate rewards, you also earn some immediate ones as well. A walk today makes you feel better *today*. Once you decide this is a turning point in your life's health, getting started is easy. And once the interest payments start rolling in (we're talking Big Benefits), who'd want to quit?

Record Meals and Snacks

SUNDAY

MONDAY

TUESDAY

WEDNESDAY

THURSDAY

FRIDAY

SATURDAY

PRACTICE DIARY THREE

Practices

Practices	Day							Notes
	Su	M	Tu	W	Th	F	Sa	
Aerobicize Your Schedule								
Skimp on Salt								
Refocus on Fiber								
3–6 servings whole grains per day								
4 servings cooked dried beans per week								
2 servings fruit per day								
3 servings vegetables per day								

✓ = yes, I did try;　　✓✓ = yes, I did welll

Suggested Practices

- Create a Clean-Air Contract to stop smoking—there's no better time.
- List immediate and lasting benefits of physical activity in One Look Back, Full Speed Ahead.
- Determine your optimum and maximum conditioning heart rate in Be Heart Smart.
- Comfort Equals Safety: warm up, stretch, cool down, and drink plenty of water when you work out.

- Take the Fitness Walking Test and determine your fitness level.
- Walk It Off: calculate your walking speed plus calories and fat-pounds burned during a typical workout week.
- Eat plenty of Fuel-Efficient Carbos (complex carbohydrates) for energy.
- Record your meals and snacks for one or more days this week in the space provided here.

WEEK FOUR

Quality Control Assurance
    The Good Food Guide
    Inside the Good Food Guide
    *Counting Burgers, Beans, and Bananas
    Deceiving Calories
    Portion Practice
    Practice: Rely on the Good Food Guide

Living Lean with *Less* Protein
    *Personalized Protein Prescription
    Practice: Moderate Your Meat Intake

*Practice Diary Four

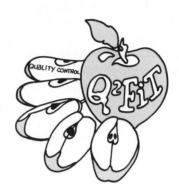

Quality Control Assurance

The Nutrition Checkup in Chapter 2 implies we need to select our foods from several different food groups every day. But some of the foods in each group are nutritionally superior to the others, a fact often obscured by glitzy TV advertisements and all-you-can-eat promotions. To make certain you are not adrift in a sea of culinary confusion, battered about by a whirlwind of relentless food ad campaigns, the Good Food Guide is here to serve as a point of reference—your nutritional North Star.

If you select your foods primarily from the Good Food Guide, you can be assured you are boosting your nutritional status by practicing Quality Control. And when you succeed in eating the minimum recommended number of choices from each food group, you may also be less hungry for high-calorie, low-nutrient sweets, alcohol, and fried foods. So the Good Food Guide works for Quantity Control, too. The guide is one of the easiest ways to estimate what and how much you do eat, or what and how much you should eat, without the drudgery of counting calories.

The Good Food Guide is divided into six major food groups: Whole Grain/ Starch, Protein, Vegetable, Fruit, Milk, and Fat. For each food group, the guide shows the amount of food that is considered 1 portion, along with the approximate number of calories and grams of protein, carbohydrate, and fat per portion. If you eat double the amount listed—two slices of bread instead of one, for example—you are eating 2 portions. The portion sizes are typical of what you would encounter at a restaurant, except for Protein (1 portion equals *1* ounce of meat).

Use the accompanying nutrition information to compare calories within and between food groups and to identify good protein or carbohydrate foods or foods likely to contain hidden fat. Complex carbohydrate in whole grain bread, cereal, pasta, rice, and starches like corn, peas, and potatoes provides sustained energy as well as filling dietary fiber; simple carbohydrate in fruits is a good source of quick energy. Protein foods like meat, cheese, eggs, milk, and yogurt are used to build and repair body tissue, while protein and fat in foods make a meal satisfying and keep you from getting hungry again so soon.

Notice, too, the Whole Grain/Starch, Vegetable, and Fruit lists sport a check mark (✓) because they are high-fiber foods you should emphasize. (Cooked dried beans in the Protein list also have dietary fiber.) The Protein and Fat lists are marked with a dollar sign ($) because they carry a high calorie cost from obvious and hidden fats, and choices from these lists should be monitored carefully. (Whole milk is another $ food.)

As an informed adult eater, you have a number of options for your Living Lean project, and one of them is to skip the Training Table plans and menus found in Chapter 6. Instead, simply use this Good Food Guide as a reference when you shop, cook, and eat. Many Living Lean participants choose this route, and it works well when you add support from the rest of the Success Formula, especially Fitness (Chapter 3) and Timing (Chapter 2). Do keep one eye on the suggested minimum number of servings for each food group to maintain Quality Control. Another helpful resource is the inventory of Outstanding Fiber Foods in Chapter 2. With the Good Food Guide, you no longer have to concentrate on a long list of things not to eat. Instead, focus on things *to* eat—choose *more*.

Now spend some time getting acquainted with the detailed Good Food Guide lists.

THE GOOD FOOD GUIDE

✓ **Whole Grain/Starch:** 80 calories; minimum 5 portions recommended daily

carbohydrate	15 grams
protein	3 grams

1 slice or 1-ounce piece whole grain* bread
1 whole grain biscuit**, muffin**, roll, tortilla, or waffle**
2 whole grain bread sticks, brown rice cakes, or pancakes**; 2-inch cube whole grain corn bread**
½ whole grain bun, bagel, English muffin, or pita bread
½ cup whole grain pasta or cooked cereal grains
⅓ cup cooked barley, brown rice, or sweet potato; ⅓ cup cooked dried beans or peas†
¾ cup whole grain dry cereal; 1½ cups whole grain puffed cereal
½ cup fresh corn, lima beans, mashed potatoes, peas, or winter squash; 1 *small* baked potato, 1 ear of corn
3 tablespoons whole grain flour or cornmeal; 2 tablespoons cornstarch or tapioca
¾ ounce (2–4) whole grain crackers or pretzels (fat-free)
3 cups air-popped popcorn, without added butter
1 cup whole grain croutons, low-fat; ¼ cup whole grain bread stuffing**

*Whole grains are always the preferred choice, but many times they aren't available, so substitute refined flour products.

**Count an additional 1 Fat portion for the fat cooked into breads like biscuits and pancakes. Butter or gravy spread or ladled over them counts *extra*.

†For larger portions of beans or peas, refer to the Protein list.

$ **Protein:** 75 calories; minimum 3 portions (women) or 4 portions (men) recommended daily

protein	7 grams
fat	5 grams

1 ounce lean beef*, pork*, lamb*, fish*, or poultry* (without skin)
2 ounces crab*, lobster*, shrimp*, or scallops*

6 oysters*; 2 sardines*

1 ounce (1-inch cube) low-fat cheese, like part-skim mozzarella

1 ounce extra-lean lunch meat* (95% fat-free)

¼ cup (4 tablespoons) cottage cheese* (dry curd or low-fat), ricotta cheese (part-skim), salmon or tuna* (packed in water)

1 egg; or 2 egg whites plus ½–1 teaspoon oil

2 tablespoons grated Parmesan cheese; 3 tablespoons grated low-fat cheese or cooked lean ground round*

1 cup cooked dried beans or peas*†

3–4 ounces tofu

2 tablespoons sesame seeds‡, sunflower seeds‡, pumpkin seeds‡, brewer's yeast; 1 tablespoon peanut butter‡

*Proteins marked with an asterisk (*) were chosen from the Lean Protein List found later in this chapter. Items on this list average only 55 calories per portion (but some choices, like low-fat seafood, may have as few as 25 calories); 2 Lean List portions equal 1 Fat portion in saved calories, so treat yourself to an extra Fat portion if you like.

†Count an additional 2 Grain/Starch portions (for ½ cup, count as ½ Protein plus 1 Grain/Starch).

‡Count an additional 1 Fat portion.

✓ **Vegetable:** 25 calories; minimum 3 portions recommended daily

carbohydrate	5 grams
protein	2 grams

½ cup cooked vegetable or vegetable juice

1 cup salad or raw vegetable

2 tablespoons tomato paste, ⅓ cup tomato sauce

1 large tomato

✓ **Fruit:** 60 calories; minimum 2 portions recommended daily

carbohydrate	15 grams

1 piece fruit

½ cup fruit or juice (unsweetened)

1 cup berries, melon, or papaya

12 grapes or cherries; ½ large banana, ½ cup sliced bananas

2 pieces or ¼ cup dried fruit

2 tablespoons raisins

✓ **Milk:** 90 calories (skim) to 120 calories (low-fat); 2 portions recommended daily

carbohydrate	12 grams
protein	8 grams
fat	5 grams (low-fat)

1 cup skim (0% fat) or nearly skim (½%, 1% fat) milk, yogurt, or buttermilk

1 cup low-fat (1½%, 2%) milk, yogurt, or buttermilk

5 tablespoons or ⅓ cup nonfat dry milk

$ **Fat:** 45 calories; minimum 3 portions recommended daily*

fat	5 grams

1 teaspoon oil, mayonnaise, margarine, or *butter;* 1 pat margarine or *butter*

1 tablespoon salad dressing, reduced-calorie mayonnaise or margarine (check the calorie label), regular or Neufchatel "light" *cream cheese*

2 tablespoons reduced-calorie salad dressing (check the calorie label) or *sour cream*

5 large or 10 small olives

⅛ or 1 ounce avocado; 2 tablespoons guacamole (mashed avocado)

1 tablespoon sunflower seeds, pumpkin seeds, sesame seeds, or chopped nuts; ½ tablespoon sesame tahini

4 pecan or walnut halves; 6 almonds

10 large or 20 small peanuts

*Fat intake from all sources—Protein, Milk, Fat, Hidden Fat, and Extras—should be a *maximum* of 5 to 6 grams per 200 calories, or 20 to 30 percent of total calories. Saturated fats are in italics.

$ Hidden Fat

Count 1 additional Fat portion for each item listed below:

2 ounces beef or pork ribs, rib roast or steak, brisket, regular hamburger, sausage, cold cuts, Prime cuts of meat, any fatty meat, most restaurant meats

2 ounces cheese, including American, Cheddar, Swiss, brie, most others

1 ounce fatty meat plus 1 ounce regular cheese

1 cup whole milk; 2 cups 2½% milk

1 fried or scrambled egg; 1 slice bacon; 1 hot dog (chicken or turkey)

1 biscuit, muffin, waffle, or matzo ball

2 pancakes, potato pancakes, or taco shells; 2-inch cube corn bread

1 ounce (4–6) crackers with fat as an ingredient (3–5 grams fat or more per serving)

2 cups oil-popped or microwave popcorn, no added butter

10 french fries; 7 potato chips; 4 tortilla chips (½ ounce or ½ cup most chips)

¼ cup granola or bread stuffing

½ cup chow mein noodles, buttered vegetables, or fried rice

1 cup stir-fried vegetables or cream soup

2 tablespoons gravy, cream sauce, onion dip, sour cream dip, or grated coconut

1 tablespoon cream cheese dip, goose liver pâté, or hollandaise sauce

1 teaspoon (5 grams) oil, mayonnaise, butter, shortening, or visible grease drizzled over or cooked into foods like fried or sauteed vegetables (fried onion rings, sauteed mushrooms), vegetables in cheese or white sauce (scalloped potatoes), bread or pastry (croissants, doughnuts), batter-fried meats (fried chicken), or broiled and basted meats (fish broiled in butter sauce)

Count 2 additional Fat portions for each item listed below:

1 hot dog (beef or pork)

½ cup potato, egg, chicken, or tuna salad or coleslaw made with regular mayonnaise

½ cup hashed brown potatoes or spinach soufflé

4 onion rings; 14 potato chips; 8 tortilla chips (1 ounce or 1 cup most chips)

1 small croissant (1½ ounces)

$ Extras

Beverages for Special Occasions

	Serving Size	Portions
Regular beer	12 ounces	3½ Fat (or 2 Fat, 1 Grain/Starch)
Light beer	12 ounces	2 Fat
Low-alcohol beer	11 ounces	1 Grain/Starch
Liquor	1½ ounces	2 Fat
Wine, dry	4 ounces	2 Fat
Wine cooler	12 ounces	3 Fat, 1 Fruit
Soft drink	12 ounces	3½ Fat
Fruit drink or lemonade	8 ounces	2½ Fat

Treats for Special Occasions*	Serving Size	Portions
Ice milk	½ cup	2 Fat (or 1 Fat, ½ Grain/Starch)
Ice cream	½ cup	3 Fat (or 2 Fat, ½ Grain/Starch)
Frozen yogurt	½ cup	1 Fat, ½ Fruit, ½ Milk (or ½ Fat, 1 Fruit, ½ Milk)
Fruit yogurt	1 cup	1½ Fat, ½ Fruit, 1½ Milk
Fruit gelatin	½ cup	1½ Fat (or 1 Fruit)
Popsicle	1 stick (1½ ounces)	1 Fat (or 1 Fruit)
Regular pudding, rice pudding, tapioca pudding	½ cup	1 Fat, ½ Grain/Starch, ½ Milk
Baked custard	½ cup	1½ Fat, ½ Grain/Starch, ½ Milk
Eggnog	½ cup	2 Fat, ½ Grain/Starch, ½ Milk
Plain cupcake	1	1 Fat, 1 Grain/Starch
Plain cake	equal to 1½ or 2 cupcakes	2 Fat, 2 Grain/Starch
with icing		add 1 Fat
Cookies	2 small (1¾ in. across)	1 Fat, 1 Grain/Starch
Vanilla wafers	3	½ Fat, ½ Grain/Starch
Granola bar or brownie	1	1 Fat, 1 Grain/Starch
Doughnut	1	2 Fat, 1½ Grain/Starch
Graham crackers	1½ (2½ in. square)	½ Grain/Starch
Animal crackers	4	½ Grain/Starch
Cranberry sauce or apple butter (unsweetened)	1 tablespoon (26–33 calories)	½ Fruit
Carob powder	2 tablespoons (30 calories)	½ Fruit
Molasses, sugar, thin chocolate syrup	1 tablespoon (43 calories)	1 Fat (or ½ Fruit)
Fruit spread (unsweetened or low-sugar)	1 tablespoon (21–42 calories)	½ Fruit
Jam or jelly	1 tablespoon (52 calories)	1 Fat (or 1 Fruit)
Pancake syrup, honey	1 tablespoon (61 calories)	1½ Fat (or 1 Fruit)
Pancake syrup, reduced-calorie	1 tablespoon (25–50 calories)	½ to 1 Fat (or ½ to 1 Fruit)
Candy, any type	1 ounce	2½ Fat (or 1 Fat, 1 Fruit)
Candy bar	1 ounce	3½ Fat (or 2 Fat, 1 Fruit)

*Treats not listed include pies and patty shells (3½ to 4 Fat portions), cheesecake and carrot cake with cream cheese frosting (4 to 5 Fat portions), and pecan pie (5 to 6 Fat portions). Unlike the above Extras list, however, these values *don't* account for sugar.

INSIDE THE GOOD FOOD GUIDE

Whole Grain/Starch

In the old days, bread and starches were on the "avoid" list because carbohydrates were thought to be fattening. Now with high-fiber whole grains as our standard and white flour products as the exception, the tables are turned. Whole grain bread, cereal, pasta, and starchy vegetables like potatoes, peas, and corn are preferred choices for Living Lean (but watch out for the cheese, butter, and sour cream that often smother them).

The suggested minimum of 5 portions a day from this list may be a departure from your usual eating routine, but it doesn't mean you have to eat five pieces of bread every day; instead, enjoy the variety in this food group. For example, one sandwich (2 portions), a small baked potato (1 portion), and two-thirds cup of rice (2 portions) would easily fill the bill. If you have trouble eating enough of these foods during the day, try adding brown rice, sweet potatoes, or dried beans to the menu—one cup is worth 3 Grain/Starch portions.

If you are attempting to cut down on meat (see Moderate Your Meat Intake), begin thinking of dried beans as a major protein source instead of just a side dish. In small amounts (say, one-third cup) you would count dried beans as a Grain/Starch portion. For larger amounts, refer to the Protein food list.

🫙 LABEL LINGO

The label should be your ultimate clue to portion size, since the foods you purchase may not be equivalent to those listed in the Good Food Guide. If your small brown rice crackers are only 7 calories each, for example, a dozen crackers would equal 84 calories, or 1 Grain/Starch portion. Should you encounter unlabeled mystery breads at the deli, just weigh out 1 ounce and you have 1 portion. (For drier grains like crackers, 3/4 ounce is closer to 1 portion.)

Handy Measures
16 tablespoons = 8 ounces = 1 cup
2 tablespoons = 1 ounce
1 tablespoon = 1/2 ounce = 3 teaspoons

Protein

Since a Protein portion consists of only 1 ounce of cheese or meat, a 6-ounce serving of roast beef would equal 6 Protein portions (and watch as your protein allowance for the day disappears in a wink). The only way to consistently live lean is to cut the size of meat portions and plan some meatless meals. A serving of 1 or 2 ounces of chicken won't be satisfying for a hungry person unless it's stretched by combining it with noodles, rice, or vegetables. However, you *will* find cooked dried beans and tofu quite filling, even in 1- or 2-portion amounts.

Most all protein foods contain some fat, an additional reason to shrink your serving size. Cooked dried beans, an excellent stand-in for meat, are a notable exception. Ditto for dry-curd cottage cheese, one of the few truly low-fat cheeses (less than 3 grams of fat, or less than 55 calories per ounce). If you're in the market for a moderate fat cheese (less than 5 grams of fat or 75 calories per ounce), try those made with part-skim milk, like mozzarella, or special reduced-calorie cheeses. Brands vary, so be sure to check labels.

If you want to create a "lean list" for your Protein foods, here are some good choices, arranged roughly in order of increasing fat:

Lean Protein List

Cooked dried beans and peas
Pot or cottage cheese, especially dry
  curd and 1% fat
Wild game
Most seafood
Veal, except for cutlets

Poultry without skin, especially white
  meat
Select grade beef loin, round, and flank
Lean ham (pork or turkey), Canadian
  bacon, 95% fat-free lunch meat, and
  pork tenderloin

SIZING UP MEAT PORTIONS

Raw meat like hamburger or steak usually shrinks 25 percent during cooking. An 8-ounce T-bone on the menu is about 6 ounces of meat on the table.

1 ounce	= 4 medium shrimp
2 ounces	= 1 chicken leg or thigh; some fast-food burgers
3 ounces	= 1 small chicken leg and thigh; 1 small chicken breast
	= 1 medium pork chop (1/2-inch thick) with fat removed
	= 1 average hamburger
	= cooked meat the size and thickness (1/2 inch) of the palm of your hand
	= 2 thin (1/4-inch) slices roast beef (3 inches square)
4 ounces	= an average chicken breast
4 1/2 ounces	= an average pork chop or serving of beef
6 ounces	= an average steak

LABEL LINGO

Labels reveal that some lean proteins like ham, Canadian bacon, 95 percent fat-free lunch meat, "diet" cheese, and canned meats like tuna and salmon are quite high in sodium. Don't trade excess fat for excess sodium!

Vegetable

At 25 calories per portion, vegetables are ad-lib foods—the more the better! Feel free to enjoy larger portions if you wish. Try to include at least three servings a day, especially dark green, yellow, or orange selections *every* day for vitamin A. Veggies from the cabbage and pepper families (broccoli, Brussels sprouts, cabbage, bell peppers) are surprisingly rich in vitamin C. Enjoy a "C food" daily as well.

Fruit

Fruit is Nature's own snack choice—high in carbohydrate energy and potassium but low in sodium. Citrus, strawberries, and watermelon offer a good vitamin C ration; apricots and other orange-colored fruits are super vitamin A sources; and cantaloupe, mangos, and papayas have both vitamins A and C.

For small fruits like figs, plums, or tangerines, two would equal 1 portion. Apricots are low in calories, so four count as 1 portion. Use standard cafeteria helpings or reasonable servings as a guide in selecting other portion sizes—for example, one-half grapefruit or one-third cantaloupe. Choose fruit that is fresh, unsweetened, or canned in its own juice. (Even so, three-fourths cup fresh but only one-third cup canned pineapple equals 1 Fruit portion.)

Don't overdo fruit juice, grapes, or sweet dried fruits like raisins, dates, and figs. Though listed servings are interchangeable where calories are concerned, they may not offer the same staying power. (For instance, only one-third cup grape juice equals 1 Fruit portion.) When you're really hungry, go for high-volume choices: one cup of strawberries instead of a dried fig. (Dried apricots are an eat-'em-up snack, though, with seven per portion.) Feel free to eat less than a whole portion, however, for any fruit.

Milk

You might think of milk as simply a substitute for tea or water, but a glass of milk or a cup of yogurt has high-quality protein equal to an ounce of meat or cheese or to one egg. One to two cups of milk, yogurt, or buttermilk daily are suggested to boost your calcium intake. While you are drinking your toast to healthier bones, you might as well try to wean yourself off of whole milk—gradually. Start with 2½ percent fat milk, then try 2 percent fat or less. At 150 calories, each glass of full-fat milk has the equivalent of two teaspoons of butter or three tablespoons of sour cream. And if you're going to have butter, why not enjoy it on a dinner roll instead of hidden in milk? Two percent milk has 120 calories per cup, but skim milk has only 90—a substantial savings.

Fat

The Fat food group is more luxury than necessity, but a little fat adds fat-soluble vitamins and essential fatty acids. Fat also makes plain but nutritious foods more enticing and helps ward off hunger. Nuts and seeds have the edge over other fats because of their fiber and crunch appeal, and like vegetable oil, mayonnaise, avocado, and olives, they are unsaturated. Be sure to count larger amounts of sunflower, pumpkin, or sesame seeds and peanut butter as Protein-plus-Fat portions (as described in the Protein list), especially if you are a vegetarian.

For pure fats like mayonnaise, oil, shortening, butter, margarine, or the fat clinging to a piece of meat, one measuring teaspoon (5 grams) equals 1 Fat portion and approximately 45 calories. Be careful: the latest research indicates fat calories are the most fattening. A small slip of the squeeze margarine bottle can squirt a lot of extra calories on your bread or vegetables, depositing extra inches around your waistline. The right touch is a *light* touch of fat.

Hidden Fat

Besides the obvious fats in the Good Food Guide, keep a sharp eye out for hidden fats. The pat of butter you spread on your roll may catch your eye and ring up a Fat portion. But what about the butter cooked into your roll, broccoli, or potatoes? What about the shortening in the piecrust? Or the fat in the breading of your fried fish? And then there are the mayonnaise- and vinaigrette-soaked salads at the salad bar. Even if you decide not to tally your daily Fats, at least become intimately acquainted with this list. It could make the difference between living lean and living *not* so lean. The following equation is worth remembering:

1 teaspoon oil = 1 pat butter or margarine =
5 grams fat =
45 calories

CALORIE EQUIVALENTS

1 tablespoon butter, margarine, mayonnaise, or oil	=	3 tablespoons cream cheese, salad dressing, or whipped cream
		or
		6 tablespoons sour cream or avocado
		or
		18 almonds
1 tablespoon reduced-calorie margarine or mayonnaise	=	1 tablespoon *regular* salad dressing or sour cream

The message here is that butter, margarine, mayonnaise, and oil are richer in calories than other fats. However, these calorie comparisons don't take into account the negative health effects of saturated fats (all those in italics on the Fat list). And reduced-calorie versions of margarine, mayonnaise, and especially salad dressing lose Brownie points because of their high sodium content. Olives are briny, too—still more good reasons to use *all* Fat portions sparingly.

🥫 LABEL LINGO

In judging fat content, you play a guessing game whenever you eat at restaurants. But you do have access to some inside information when you're trying to decide between Brand A and Brand B at the supermarket. It's all on the nutrition label: each 45 calories from fat (or each 5 grams of fat) will count as 1 Fat or Hidden Fat portion, regardless of what the Good Food Guide says.

For example, if a package of frozen biscuits lists 7 grams of fat for one biscuit, you should allow 1½ Fat portions per biscuit instead of 1 Fat portion, as the Good Food Guide indicates. And this isn't the only convenience-food product that delivers more fat than a similar home-made product.

Extras

"I don't see Cheetos or Milky Ways on the Good Food Guide." "How do I count two frozen margaritas?" As you may have noticed, alcohol, sweets, and snack foods don't work well as staples when you're attempting to live lean. But you *can* enjoy them for special occasions and still remain in command of your Living Lean project.

In the Extras list, fat calories are always calculated as Fat portions. Sugar and alcohol calories may appear either as Fat portions or as Grain/Starch or Fruit portions. If you eat too much rich food, obviously something has to give, and fatty foods are the most expendable because they contribute so few nutrients. If you know how many calories your Extra contains, you can scratch the appropriate number of Fat portions from your daily total.

Sometimes you have to exchange a piece of fresh fruit for a spoon of jam or a whole grain muffin for a cookie, but try not to trade away more than one serving of nutritious food in a day. Otherwise, you'll end up with plenty of calories but few nutrients when you add up your totals. Limit pure sweeteners—sugar, fructose, honey, jam or jelly, syrup—to one or two teaspoons per day. Think Quality Control as well as Quantity Control.

HOME COOKING

In a home recipe, watch your salt, sugar, and fat ingredients. If the recipe calls for one-half cup sugar and serves four people, then each person gets two tablespoons of sugar. If one stick of butter is in a recipe that serves eight, you end up with one tablespoon of butter or 3 Fat portions per person.

 ## COUNTING BURGERS, BEANS, AND BANANAS

Now try your hand at using the Good Food Guide. Determine the number of portions from each food group for these dishes.

a. 1 cup brown rice with 1 pat butter _____

b. plain cheeseburger _____

c. 2 cups garden salad with 1 tablespoon dressing _____

d. 1 cup black beans _____

e. 6 pecan halves (3 whole pecans) _____

f. 1 large banana _____

g. ½ grapefruit and 2 fresh cherries _____

Answers

a. 3 Grain/Starch
   1 Fat
b. 2 Grain/Starch (bun)
   3 Protein (3 ounces meat)
   1 Protein (1 ounce cheese)
c. 2 Vegetable
   1 Fat

d. 1 Protein plus 2 Grain/Starch
e. 1½ Fat
f. 2 Fruit
g. 1 Fruit (if less than half a portion, as for cherries, ignore it)

DECEIVING CALORIES

What if you are fairly haphazard at estimating portion sizes or keeping records? Suppose you eat two cups of salad but record it as only one cup? Or you accidentally eat three-fourths cup of green beans instead of one-half cup? These mistakes are mostly to your benefit, since veggies contribute more nutrition and fiber than they do calories; and if they are omitted, some other food with more calories and less fiber and nutrition is likely to quench your appetite.

What about a Protein or Fat list food? Does the serving size make that much difference? You bet your brisket it does! One ounce of sausage has only 100 calories, but 10 ounces deliver 1,000. Remember:

Fatty meats and most cheeses = 100 calories per ounce

Calories for a typical restaurant meal might stack up as follows when analyzed with the Good Food Guide:

Number of Servings	Calories
1 cup low-fat milk	120
2 to 3 vegetables	50–75
1 fruit	60
2 starches (large potato) and 1 grain (roll)	240
5 to 8 ounces cooked high-fat meat (Prime rib)	500–800
or	or
medium-fat meat (T-bone steak)	375–600
4 to 5 added fats (butter, salad dressing, sauce)	180–225

Which foods contribute the most calories in this meal? Which foods have the most fat calories? For this meal, logging in 5 ounces of meat instead of 8 means a bottom-line error of 225 to 300 calories—a figure worth two extra baked potatoes or four additional ears of corn! Watch out for meats and cheeses—the calories can really be deceiving.

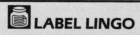

LABEL LINGO

Do you know the Label Lingo when it comes to calories?

- "Low calorie" means less than 40 calories per serving (watch that serving size) or less than 10 calories per ounce.
- "Reduced calorie" means calories are reduced by at least 33 percent.
- "Light" or "lite" could mean light in color or texture.
- "Diet" or "dietetic" may not refer to calorie content.

PORTION PRACTICE

In order to avoid eating a tablespoon of butter or 8 ounces of meat when you don't mean to, you first have to be able to recognize a tablespoon or 8 ounces when you see it. One Living Lean student would weigh a chicken breast before dinner, then weigh the bones and scraps remaining after dinner. From the difference he calculated how much he had actually eaten.

Try weighing or measuring the following portions in your kitchen, in both large and small serving dishes. Be sure to use standard measuring utensils. (Don't be like the man who used the biggest spoon in the kitchen drawer to measure his "one tablespoon of peanut butter.") Then when you encounter these dishes in a genuine meal, you'll have a mental picture of the portion size you're after.

¼ cup tuna (1½ to 2 ounces—half a small 3½-ounce can or one-fourth a standard 6½-ounce can)

2 ounces hamburger (a regular hamburger is about 3 ounces when cooked)

1 and 2 ounces roast beef, steak, and chicken

1 ounce lunch meat (most slices are ¾ ounce or less—close enough)

1 ounce cheese (a 1-inch cube or a slice of cheeseburger cheese; most wrapped slices are ¾ ounce)

2½ to 3 tablespoons grated cheese (also 1 ounce; try sprinkling it over vegetables, a potato, or a salad to get a useful mental picture)

½ cup cottage cheese (half a small 8-ounce carton)

1 tablespoon salad dressing (try this with both thick and thin dressings)

1 tablespoon peanut butter (spread on bread or crackers)

2 tablespoons raisins (a tiny ½-ounce raisin snack pack is 1½ tablespoons)

1 teaspoon butter or mayonnaise (spread on bread, a roll, or a cracker; could you be satisfied with half a teaspoon?)

6 almonds or 12 grapes (how many equal a handful for you?)

½ cup ice milk or ice cream (4 ounces or one small scoop)

FAT-SKIMMED FAVORITES

Do your health a favor—and your waistline, too—with this skinny version of brown gravy. (The brewer's yeast in this recipe isn't essential, but it does add a meaty taste.)

🥤 Low-Fat Gravy

¾ cup defatted drippings or broth and ¼ cup milk *or* 1 cup broth or stock *or* 1 cup water
2 tablespoons whole wheat pastry flour
1 low-salt bouillon cube
1 tablespoon brewer's yeast flakes
¼ teaspoon garlic powder
¼ teaspoon onion powder
¼ teaspoon thyme
¼ teaspoon salt or tamari soy sauce (omit if bouillon cube used)
⅛ teaspoon black pepper
⅛ teaspoon savory
pinch celery seeds

Stir pastry flour into liquid before heating. Add bouillon cube (if used) and seasonings, and bring to a boil, stirring constantly. Lower heat and simmer at least 12 minutes, stirring occasionally.

🥤 Breakfast Sausage

In the same time it takes to cook a hamburger, you can make this tasty sausage. Your breakfast treat will have less than 30 percent fat calories instead of 80 percent, the average for commercial sausage. You don't need loads of fat, just the right spices to deliver that familiar wake-up flavor and aroma. (And if you're experimenting with smaller meat portions this week, note that one-half recipe equals just 1½ ounces after cooking.)

2 ounces ground pork tenderloin   ¼ teaspoon black pepper
2 ounces lean ground round   ⅛ teaspoon cayenne
½ teaspoon sage   pinch thyme
¼ teaspoon marjoram   pinch nutmeg

Knead the beef and pork together along with the seasonings. Pan-fry without added fat, pouring off drippings as they accumulate. Cook on both sides until done; drain on paper towels before serving.

½ recipe = 1½ Protein

✓ PRACTICE: RELY ON THE GOOD FOOD GUIDE

Do you eat *enough* of the right foods? Let the Good Food Guide lead you toward better health: for this week, select your meals and snacks primarily (if not exclusively) from this list. Try to eat at least the suggested minimum number of portions from each food group to ensure good nutrition. (A bonus: if you eat more "good food," some of the less desirable choices may be squeezed off your menu.)

Suggested Minimum Daily Portions

Food Group	Portion Number
Grain/Starch	5–7+ (7–9+)
Protein	3–4
Vegetable	3+
Fruit	2+
Milk	2
Fat	3–5

Fill in these suggested portion numbers on the top row of the Good Food Guide Tally in the Practice Diary at the end of the chapter. (If you're an active woman or have a hefty appetite, be sure to use the 7–9+ minimum for Grain/Starch portions. If you're a man, use the greater number for each food group.) There are spaces to then record the number of Good Food Guide portions you eat for breakfast, lunch, dinner, and snacks, plus daily totals; also record any foods *not* found in the guide.

In the first example below, a woman counted 3 Hidden Fat portions for her dish of ice cream; she chose not to list portions for her candy bar. At the end of the day, she circled the food group totals that failed to meet the suggested minimum. (In her case, more veggies and milk might have reduced her ice cream-and-candy craving.) In the second example, a man is keeping track of his daily portion totals for a week, with one day per line. That way, he can see how his eating habits vary from day to day.

SAMPLE GOOD FOOD GUIDE TALLIES

ONE-DAY RECORD

Sug. Daily Por.	Gr/St	Pro	Veg	Fruit	Milk	F/HF	Extras
	7+	3	3+	2+	2	3	
B	3			2	1	1	
S							Candy Bar
L	2	2		1		2	
S	1						
D	1	3½	1				
S						(3)	Ice cream
Total	7	5½	(1)	3	(1)	6	✓✓

Sug. Daily Por. = Suggested Daily Portions
Gr/St = Grain/Starch   Veg = Vegetables
Pro = Protein   F/HF = Fat/Hidden Fat

SEVEN-DAY RECORD

Sug. Daily Por.	Gr/St	Pro	Veg	Fruit	Milk	F/HF	Extras
	9+	4	3+	3+	2	5	
Su	⦸⦸ ///	⦸⦸ ///	////	///	//	⦸⦸ //	
M	⦸⦸ /	////	///	⦸⦸	/	⦸⦸ /	//
Tu							
W							
Th							
F							
Sa							

Sug. Daily Por. = Suggested Daily Portions
Gr/St = Grain/Starch   Veg = Vegetables
Pro = Protein   F/HF = Fat/Hidden Fat

If you're like most folks, you'll discover it's easy to eat the minimum Protein and Fat portions—perhaps *too* easy. If so, opt for more fiber foods from the Vegetable and Whole Grain/Starch groups, with extra Fruit portions if you need them. Whatever you do, don't go hungry; these recommendations are minimums, not maximums (except for Milk—the recommendation is both minimum *and* maximum). Remind yourself that high-fiber carbohydrates are filling, not fattening. And instead of fretting about eating too much this week, concentrate on eating *enough*. Choose more "good food" for Quality Control.

VERY GOOD VEGGIES

Do you have a hard time eating a minimum of 3 Vegetable portions every day? If so, tempt yourself by adding a brand new taste to your old standbys.

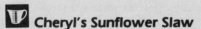 Cheryl's Sunflower Slaw

1 1/2 cups shredded cabbage
1 cup shredded carrots
1/2 cup plain low-fat yogurt
2 tablespoons sunflower seeds

2 tablespoons raisins
3/4 teaspoon red wine vinegar
1/8 teaspoon paprika
sprinkle garlic

Combine all ingredients and mix well.

1/2 cup = 1 1/2 Vegetable, 1/2 Fat

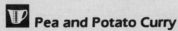 Pea and Potato Curry

Create your own convenience veggies: freeze a double batch of this curry in single-serving containers.

1 cup diced potatoes
1 cup small broccoli pieces, fresh or frozen
1 cup small cauliflower pieces, fresh or frozen

> $^1/_2$ cup green peas, fresh or frozen
> 1 tablespoon sesame oil
> $^1/_2$ cup diced onion
> 1 tablespoon lemon juice
> 1 tablespoon sesame seeds
> $^1/_2$ to $^3/_4$ teaspoon fresh curry powder
> $^1/_8$ to $^1/_4$ teaspoon ginger
> $^1/_8$ teaspoon cinnamon
> 1 cup plain low-fat yogurt (optional)
>
> Steam raw vegetables until just tender. In a wok or skillet, saute onion, lemon juice, seeds, and spices in oil until the onion is translucent. Add steamed and frozen vegetables, and stir occasionally until heated through. Serve with yogurt if you wish.
>
> $^1/_2$ recipe (1$^1/_2$ cups) = 1 Grain/Starch, 2 Vegetable, 2 Fat
>
> $^1/_2$ cup yogurt = $^1/_2$ Milk

Living Lean with *Less* Protein

How do you make a fat rat? Order him the Dieter's Delight—a dry meat patty and cottage cheese, with a tiny piece of toast. Crazy as it sounds, too much protein, the traditional "diet" food, may promote an increase rather than a decrease in body fat. When rats were fed exactly the same number of calories, but either a large or small amount of protein, the high-pro rats ended up with almost twice as much body fat. And more than 30 years ago, a group of overfat volunteers successfully lost excess pounds by eating a minimal amount of food protein but an unrestricted number of calories.

Is protein, then, more fattening than carbohydrate? This is a possibility, according to a Kentucky State University research study. The main difference researchers found in comparing the eating habits of overfat women and lean women was protein consumption: the overfat women ate more meat and milk. Carbohydrates cause more calorie burn-off after meals than do proteins, which may partly explain the consequences. Meat and dairy products are also major purveyors of hidden fat.

Since most protein fiends eat excess animal protein, it is possible that *vegetable* protein, with its attendant dietary fiber, may not share the guilt equally. In fact, vegetarians do appear to be leaner. In one survey, vegetarian men weighed 30 pounds less and vegetarian women 24 pounds less—an average 143 and 121 pounds, respectively—than their meat-eating counterparts. (The average U.S. male is 5 feet 9½ inches and weighs 173 pounds; the average female is 5 feet 4 inches and weighs 142 pounds.) Other inquiries find less spectacular differences between the veggies and the carnivores, but they usually do reveal a gap. Considering the number of Living Lean students who attribute some or all of their fat loss to a change in meat-eating habits, the subject warrants more investigation.

"But wouldn't it be risky to do without the hearty protein staple?" Not if you eat a variety of foods with protein from the Good Food Guide along with sufficient calories (i.e., no crash diets—they cause protein loss regardless of the amount of protein eaten). Even the shy foods on your plate—vegetables, salad, bread, cereal, rice, dried beans, nuts, and seeds—are willing contributors to your daily protein quota. Plus 9 out of 10 vegetarians eat high-protein cheese, milk, and eggs. Only fruits and fats are truly protein-poor.

You can figure the approximate protein offering from these various foods, and your typical intake, by checking with the Good Food Guide. Who would have thought an innocent-looking cup of broccoli, green peas, or Brussels sprouts would have almost as much protein as an egg or an ounce of cheese? You can also use the numbers to determine whether you are eating proportionately more protein from plant foods than from animal foods each day (the most recent health-maintenance recommendation).

Although it's not essential, you can elect to combine nonmeat proteins (see the Protein Pyramid) to create dishes that approximate the protein quality of meat. Bean-plus-grain favorites include red beans and rice, pinto beans and tortillas, black-eyed peas and corn bread, lentils and rice, and peanut butter and crackers. Even a small amount of high-quality animal or soy protein (like fish, yogurt, beef, egg, or tofu) will boost the quality of any plant protein you eat with it. Chicken noodle soup, macaroni and cheese, corn flakes in milk, and tofu with brown rice are just a few ways to stretch your food dollar and your protein-calorie investment as well.

There remains only one legitimate drawback to totally scratching meat from the menu: its nutritional value. Poultry and seafood contribute vitamin B_6, pork is a rich source of thiamin, and beef contains highly absorbable iron, zinc, and manganese—trace minerals in short supply even for meat eaters. Dairy products won't take up the slack for iron; in fact, the dairy-loving "dieter" is especially susceptible to "yogurt anemia" as calories shrink. Luckily, vitamin C foods can boost iron absorption from dried beans, whole grains, seeds, and vegetables, while brewer's yeast, cheese, and tofu are fairly reliable sources of zinc. Getting enough manganese is more of a challenge without red meat, however.

Still, much of the world's population eats little meat. Where food is abundant, their health statistics are enviable. The typical dairy-vegetarian diet has twice as much dietary fiber as the usual macho-meat diet. As a group, nonmeat eaters have

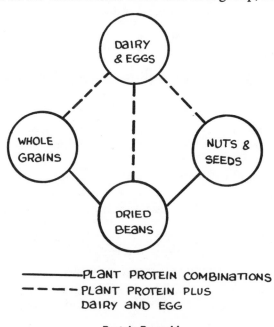

Protein Pyramid

lower blood pressure and blood cholesterol, a reduced risk of colon cancer, and half the risk of diabetes; they are leaner and they live longer. The men have three times less heart disease, and women have less osteoporosis and breast cancer.

If you're a confirmed carnivore, however, don't despair. Cutting down on meat could be healthier than cutting it out, especially if you fill in the gaps with plant foods that are typically low in calories, fat, and saturated fat. The switch can be pretty simple, too—just eat one piece of chicken instead of two, or chili with beans instead of ground beef, or more pasta and tomato sauce meals and fewer eat-and-run burgers.

✎ PERSONALIZED PROTEIN PRESCRIPTION

How much protein should you eat? According to the Recommended Dietary Allowance (which is very generous), women need 44 grams a day, and men, 56 grams a day. But women regularly eat as much as 70 grams, while men scarf down 100 grams a day or more. Your protein need is proportional to your body lean, so if your extra pounds are fat rather than muscle, your roast beef requirement isn't any greater. (Remember, excess protein equals excess calories.) In moderation, protein helps to fight hunger, so be sure to distribute your Protein portions throughout the day rather than piling them up at dinnertime.

Here's how to figure out a more personalized protein recommendation. First calculate your weight for height.

1. For men: write down 106.
   For women: write down 100.

   1. _100_

2. For men: add 6 for each inch in height above 5 feet
   For women: add 5 for each inch in height above 5 feet

   2. _20_
   weight for height

Now calculate your protein requirement. Multiply by the higher number if you are doing lots of intense muscle work or hard training.

weight for height: _120_ × .36 or .54 = _21_ grams of protein per day

_120_
_.36_
_728_
_1400_

✔ PRACTICE: MODERATE YOUR MEAT INTAKE

_21.20_

Your Paleolithic cousins weren't vegetarians. In fact, they ate meat in mammoth amounts. But before you honor your ancestors with a 12-ounce T-bone, consider this: their wild game was lower in fat than anything you can buy in a butcher shop today.

If you typically eat to the primitive beat (that is, lots of meat), this week trade your hunter's bow for a gatherer's basket. Limit your meat servings (beef, pork, chicken, fish) to 1 to 3 ounces. Try to eat meat only once a day, and a couple of days not at all.

If you're not bullish on meat, chances are you're hooked on cheese. Unfortunately regular cheese has as much fat as fatty meats like hot dogs, sausage, and ribs, so perform the same reduction ritual with cheese, only limit servings to ½ to 1 ounce. For a *real* challenge, you might also try to eat no more than 3 (women) or 4 (men) Protein portions each day this week. You'll still get plenty of protein when you add in the other food groups.

Next time you forage through the supermarket aisles, consider the rumblings from your stomach to be compelling echoes from ancient drums. The message? Gather most of your groceries from high-fiber produce bins, grain shelves, and legume racks, with just a quick stop at the dairy case; and cut your hunting time in the low-fiber meat department in half.

✏️ ✓ Practice Diary Four

Have you been consistently working out and eating right thus far? If the answer is "yes," congratulations—because by this week you should start to see some fat reduction (in inches) even if your weight is not yet changing.

But be prepared. In spite of the good news, you are still likely to hit a psychological slump along about now, when the novelty of Living Lean wears off and the reality sets in. There is always a little sadness with any goodbye; but as you let go of the old, unproductive habits to make room for the new ones, you will round an important turning point to find more self-confidence and renewed enthusiasm the second four weeks.

And why not? By staying active and choosing your foods primarily from the Good Food Guide, you can accomplish Quality and Quantity Control in eating, without resorting to calorie counting or extreme restrictions. As has been said before, the Success Formula really works—you can *count* on it.

RECORD MEALS AND SNACKS

SUNDAY

MONDAY

TUESDAY

WEDNESDAY

THURSDAY

FRIDAY

SATURDAY

PRACTICE DIARY FOUR

Practices

	Day							Notes
	Su	M	Tu	W	Th	F	Sa	
Aerobic Activity—30 minutes, 4 days a week								
Rely on the Good Food Guide								
Moderate Your Meat Intake								

✓ = yes, I did try;   ✓✓ = yes, I did well!

Suggested Practices

■ Choose proteins primarily from the Lean Protein List.

■ Recognize typical meat servings in Sizing Up Meat Portions.

■ Monitor each person's share of sugar, salt, and fat in the Home Cooking recipes.

■ Weigh and measure the foods you eat often in Portion Practice.

GOOD FOOD GUIDE TALLY

	Gr/St	Pro	Veg	Fruit	Milk	F/HF	Extras
Sug. Daily Por.							

Sug. Daily Por. = Suggested Daily Portions (Minimum)
Gr/St = Grain/Starch   Veg = Vegetables
Pro = Protein   F/HF = Fat/Hidden Fat

WEEK FIVE

Meet Your Metabolism
    Why Successful "Diets" Can Fail
    What You See Is (Not Necessarily) What You Get
    Reset the Setpoint
    Activity Aids Appropriate Appetite
    Where Do the Calories Go?

Fitness: Beyond Good Intentions
    *Hurdling Aerobic Obstacles
    Be an Activist!
    *Choose to Move
    *Activity Log: A Day in the Life
    Practice: Swing into Action
    *Practice: Personal Time Out

Sticks and Stones and Sturdy Bones
    *Count on Calcium
    Strong Women

*Practice Diary Five

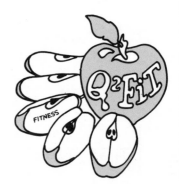

Meet Your Metabolism

Sigh. "I could live on salads and cottage cheese and still gain weight. I just have a slow metabolism, I guess." Ah, the typical cop-out of the weak-willed dieter, right? Not necessarily.

Suppose you see two women sitting side by side on a park bench. Both weigh 140 pounds, though one is quite lean and the other has a substantial amount of body fat. If they are sharing a box lunch, which one should get more food? (In other words, which one has a faster metabolism, or rate of calorie burning?) Calorie requirement is proportional to the amount of lean muscle each woman has, among other things. Fat needs fewer calories to maintain it; basically, it just sits there. So the lean woman gets a little more chicken—and the biscuit.

Muscle is your calorie-burning factory, so to speak. Mitochondria (the energy powerhouse of cells) in your muscles are like heat- and energy-producing furnaces, while enzymes are the laborers stoking the furnaces with fuel. Aerobically trained muscles have more laborers and larger, more efficient furnaces than do untrained, weak muscles. And the furnaces are better adapted to burning fat for fuel—not only while you're swimming laps, but also later on when you're pitching horseshoes or just sitting and knitting. "So how can I get more of this fat-burning muscle?"

Only one way: muscles fall into the use-'em-or-lose-'em category. They shrink from disuse as we get older, one of the main reasons our metabolism slows from 2 to 5 percent every 10 years—enough to account for 25 of our additional fat-pounds by the time we hit 60. And these changes in body composition can occur even with little or no change in body weight, as the graph shows. Women theoretically have

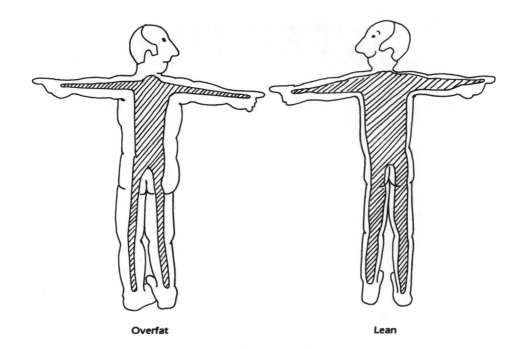

Overfat   Lean

slower metabolic rates than men because they have more fat and less muscle. But a lean, athletic woman might require just as much food as an out-of-shape male her same size.

Even if you're not "athletic," physical activity is a great way to increase metabolic output from muscles you already have. For one thing, your metabolism remains in higher gear (burning more calories) anywhere from an hour to a day or more after a strenuous workout. Physical effort also sends a message to build more muscle, making your factory bigger and thus more productive. The bottom line is increased calorie combustion, making it easier to stay lean even in the face of inevitable eating excesses. For Living Lean purposes, *mighty muscle means maximum metabolism.*

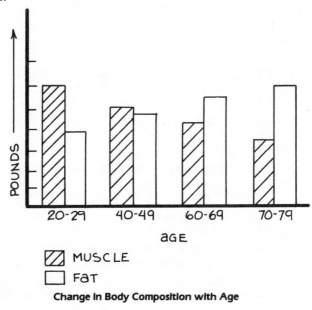

Change in Body Composition with Age

WHY SUCCESSFUL "DIETS" CAN FAIL

Because eating excesses are common, most people figure the easiest way to lose weight is to eat less. But beware of taking in substantially less food than your body needs; in addition to the misleading initial glycogen and water weight loss described in Chapter 1, a low-calorie "diet" can really foul up your metabolism, perhaps for a good long time.

For instance, when you gain weight without aerobic sweat, it's mostly fat (as much as 70 to 100 percent). But when you lose it by "dieting," anywhere from 25 to 75 percent may be lean muscle, sacrificed for an additional source of calories. (From your body's point of view, energy needs are more important than muscle that isn't being used much anyway.) When lean disappears, you can bid farewell to a portion of your much-needed calorie-burning factory. It doesn't take a math whiz to see that repeated "diets" can alter your lean-to-fat ratio in the wrong direction, setting you up for a rebound fat gain if the shift isn't repaired.

Aerobic activity, on the other hand, seems to protect lean (or at least minimize lean loss) during a "diet." It also helps rebuild any lost muscle, but only if you have 400 extra calories, 15 spare grams of protein, and plenty of muscle-stressing activity every day. Even at that rate, you can only make about a pound of new muscle a week.

Should you opt for a "diet" of less than 1,200 calories, however, you may lose your lean in spite of diligent physical activity. For example, a 1,000-calorie diet study produced weight loss that was 12 percent lean the second week and 15 percent lean by the fourth week, even with two and a half hours of daily exercise.

More bad news: with or without the muscle loss, metabolism is still likely to decline with traditional "dieting." When lean, active men initiated a 1,600-calorie regimen, their metabolic rates plummeted 50 percent. The same slowdown occurred when a 38-year-old woman dropped her food calories from 2,800 to 1,000. At Ohio State University, overfat women who lost weight for several months on 420 calories a day failed to *keep* losing weight when their calories were increased only to 800, partly because their metabolic rates had fallen by 355 calories a day. Another group of overfat males were semistarved on 450 calories a day, and their collective resting metabolism fell to match. As illustrated, weight loss slowed to a virtual halt in less than a month.

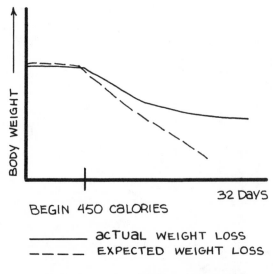

Weight Loss with a Very Low Calorie Diet

Even more discouraging, metabolism slowed by "dieting" may not fully recover when the "diet" ends. English women who successfully "dieted" down to 135 pounds and stayed there a couple of years had only slightly less lean muscle but 15 percent lower metabolic rates than women the same height and weight who had never "dieted." The "dieters" also burned fewer calories, even doing exactly the same type of physical activity. And what's worse, they were forced to maintain their 135 pounds on only 1,300 calories a day, while the "no diet" women maintained their 135 pounds on 1,985 calories a day—almost 700 calories more.

"Dieting" may also pose an insidious threat to maintenance metabolism. Volunteers who ate 500 calories less than usual were observed to spontaneously spend less time standing and walking and more time sitting. For those already moving at a pokey pace, eating less could be a shove into absolute inertia.

"So what?" you might be thinking after hearing all the evidence. "I'd still lose *weight* on a diet, and I'll never miss that dear-departed muscle. Besides, what's the worst that could happen?"

Well, you might find yourself stuck on a more or less permanent metabolic plateau—a twilight zone where you forever plead, "I really don't eat that much—honest," as your doctor shakes her head in disbelief. How low can this plateau go? Pretty darn low. An anorexic teenager maintained her weight on a plain potato, three diet drinks, a banana, and some raisins every day, even in the face of grueling swim-team workouts. A 275-pound "professional dieter" found he had to eat less than 1,000 calories a day to keep from gaining. And a 26-year-old became nearly frantic after four years of "diets" and diet pills

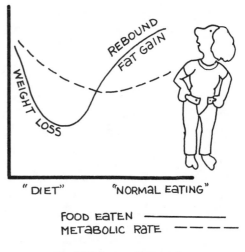

FOOD EATEN ——————
METABOLIC RATE — — — —

The Weight Loss Rebound

caught up with her. When she finally visited a dietitian, she was sustaining her "ideal weight" of 135 pounds on 590 calories a day. Even with the best of intentions, imprudent "dieting" can wreak severe metabolic damage.

For most folks, however, perpetual "dieting" is not an option. Whether the "diet" life expectancy is two weeks or two years, they ultimately abandon the restrictions only to discover something about them has changed; they now accrue fat on what was once a conservative calorie intake, as shown in the illustration. Laura, a friend of a friend, is a sad example.

After some discussion, she chose to enroll in one of the medical "diet" clinics rather than Living Lean. They offered a "pounds off or money back" guarantee, while Living Lean offered only inspiration and information. Her "diet" was the topic when the gang gathered to socialize. "Laura has lost almost 50 pounds," they reported enviously. "But is it gone for good? And is she still healthy?" Her immediate success clouded any concern for the future. "Who cares?" they replied.

After a couple of years, Laura was once again the subject of discussion. "How is she doing?" The gang became somber and spoke in hushed tones. "You wouldn't recognize her—she's as wide as she is tall. She has gained more weight than she ever lost, and she's still growing." Laura's rebound is not the first casualty of the "diet" wars, though most are not quite so devastating. Admittedly, the bait is tempting, but be forewarned—it's a trap.

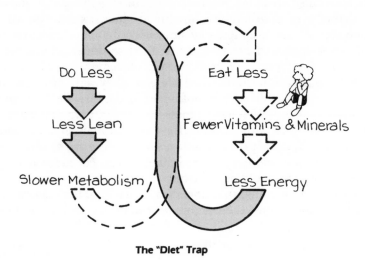

The "Diet" Trap

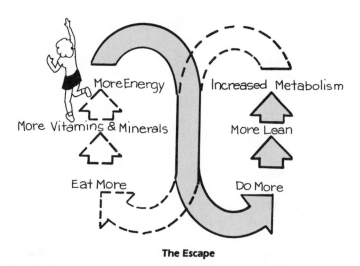

The Escape

Cutting calories—"dieting"—simultaneously diminishes your source of vitamins and minerals and your fuel for energy. You are likely to become less and less active as a result. Also, lean muscle shrinks and metabolism slows, causing an unappreciated gain in fat, even without overeating. The typical response is another "diet," and the cycle begins all over again.

Let's not hit bottom just to make a point. Break the cycle with high-quality eating and consistent aerobic effort, and you'll raise the metabolic setpoint.

Jeanne is an instructive example because she fell into the trap, and she also escaped. By her own admission "an incredibly compulsive person," Jeanne keeps running records of her weight, body measurements, food intake with calorie totals, workout miles, resting and training heart rates, and occasionally her blood glucose levels—but only when she's tuned in to her health (when she's tuned out, she exists on doughnuts and pizza).

At her most recent birthday party, she decided "slightly fat and definitely forty" weren't suited to her new self-image or her petite frame. So she pulled out a 1,200 calorie "diet" plan she uses now and then and did a couple of daily "laps" on her walking treadmill. Except this time it didn't work: no change in any of her vital statistics, including her measurements. Plus she was hungry all the time and occasionally shaky, with simultaneous low blood glucose readings. After a couple of months, she tossed the "diet" back in a drawer, and *then* things started to happen.

First of all, she began eating again. The extra energy coaxed her to stay on the treadmill a good bit longer without wilting. As time passed, it was apparent she needed even more calories than when she was a beginner treadmill walker.

The proof is in the shrinking. Not only did she lose weight eating a more reasonable amount of food, she also lost inches—a conclusive sign that her "forties" fat was giving way to "forties" fit. The shakiness eradicated, she now feels great, physically and psychologically. "What a difference a little extra food makes."

The moral of this one-woman experiment: even the best tools for determining appropriate calorie intake don't take into account changes in metabolic fitness. As you grow lean and fit, you should adjust your eating to the new and improved you. And once you have escaped the trap, make a solemn vow never to fall into it again.

WHAT YOU SEE IS (NOT NECESSARILY) WHAT YOU GET

There's another odd twist to this metabolic whodunit (or more accurately, what-dunit) that might throw you off the track, even when you're making honest progress and doing everything right. Suppose you manage a 3-pound weight loss. This loss could mean you've disposed of mostly muscle, water, and glycogen (boo, hiss), mostly fat (three cheers), or a combination of both. How do you know what's happening?

Meanwhile back at the bench, our ladies who have been breaking biscuits and nibbling on chicken both conclude they should lose some weight. The lean woman begins a swimming program, the overfat women goes on a "diet." A couple of months and thousands of incinerated calories later, the results are in. But who's the winner?

WHAT'S IN A POUND?

A fat-pound is worth about 3,500 calories; a lean- or muscle-pound, about 2,500 to 3,000 calories. Unfortunately, lean-pounds disappear more easily than they are rebuilt; and fat-pounds are created more easily than they are dismantled!

In the illustrated example on page 92, the sports enthusiast lost more fat, she lost more inches, and she looks and feels better. Plus she's boosting her metabolism and defending her fat loss with new muscle. The "diet" fan lost more weight but less fat and fewer inches; and she doesn't look or feel much different. Too, she's setting herself up for a rebound weight and fat gain by losing calorie-hungry muscle and slowing her metabolism.

Back to the question—how do you know what's really happening? Watson, Sherlock Holmes's noted sidekick, observes that aerobic activity usually protects against lean loss, which is a substantial clue; inches lost by the swimmer offer additional supporting evidence. Sherlock claims to have proof positive when the results of the ladies' fat versus lean body composition analysis are announced.

He wheels and points a finger at the culprit: our old friend, the bathroom scale, now charged "Guilty" on the basis of false and misleading testimony. Toss it

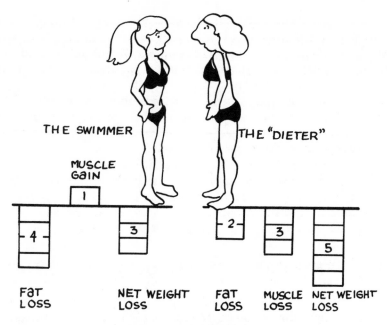

**Three Pounds vs. Five Pounds
The Winner?**

in the dungeon (or the basement if you prefer) and throw away the key. You don't need it. If you're eating healthy, working hard, feeling good, and losing inches, *you're on the right track. Keep it up!*

While this is just fiction, a genuine showdown did reveal "dieting" to be a flop due to loss of lean tissue (Group 1 in the following graph). However, when participants cut back a *little* on their customary calories (250 calories' worth), they not only lost 13 fat-pounds, they also gained a pound of muscle (Group 2). Results for Group 3, who worked off 500 calories a day but didn't alter food calories at all, were just as good or better; these folks lost 12½ fat-pounds and gained *2* pounds of muscle.

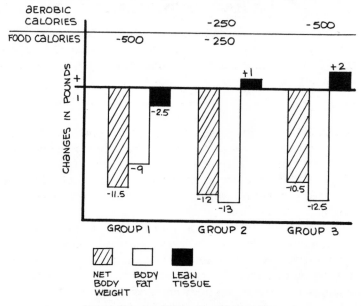

**Sixteen Weeks of Diet, Aerobic Activity,
or Both: Changes in Body Composition**

Based on a number of aerobic-only experiments similar to the Group 3 trial, a third to a half pound is the typical *weight* loss you could expect each week in exchange for reasonable aerobic effort—about 200 to 300 calories spent daily in walking four to six days a week. That's 26 scale-pounds in a year, sans "dieting." But don't forget: actual fat loss is usually greater than weight loss (both Groups 2 and 3) if you have built some new muscle in the process.

RESET THE SETPOINT

"My body constantly sabotages me into eating more than I need to." Outside of syndromes where people grow fatter seemingly without limit, this is not true or we would all be obese. On the contrary, your body has an incredible balancing mechanism, maintaining a constant body composition over time that almost defies scientific monitoring. How else do you account for a Living Lean student who weighs the same now as he did 10 years ago, when he has no bathroom scale and never learned to count calories?

For two days following a calorie orgy or fitness frenzy, your appetite and metabolism may adjust to help compensate (regrettably, persistent laziness may not invoke the same regulator

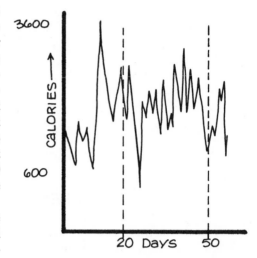

One Woman's Daily Calorie Consumption

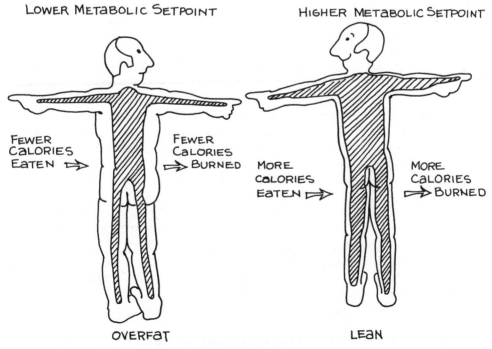

LOWER METABOLIC SETPOINT

FEWER CALORIES EATEN ⇨

FEWER CALORIES ⇨ BURNED

OVERFAT

HIGHER METABOLIC SETPOINT

MORE CALORIES EATEN ⇨

MORE CALORIES ⇨ BURNED

LEAN

Plateau Profile

mechanism). For a real challenge, try stalking a typical college student's trail of skipped meals, empty candy bar wrappers, and midnight pizza parties. In spite of on-and-off munchies like those in the preceding diagram, body weight and composition remain remarkably constant. Your eating habits may seem like a free-for-all, but there is infinite body wisdom concealed behind the consumer madness. It is up to you to uncover, dust off, and refine that balancing mechanism.

How to do it? Adopt a lean scheme that will reset your metabolic setpoint. In summary, steer clear of the "diet" trap. Loss of lean and a decline in metabolism ensure that "dieted" weight loss is rarely lost for long, and the rebound weight gain usually contains proportionately more fat. Next, raise your metabolic setpoint and lower your body fat and weight setpoint by beginning your aerobic fitness program. You may lose fat without losing weight—at first. But if you stick with your fitness goals as long as two months, lean-building will slow down and weight loss will catch up.

The infamous plateau is your body's way of expressing a preference for some status quo. Which shall it be?

Though you can't be assured of a movie star figure or a Charles Atlas physique, you can opt for a higher metabolic plateau or setpoint instead of a lower one. And if you get there the right way—using the Success Formula for Living Lean—it will be much easier to stay there. *Pick your plateau!*

ACTIVITY AIDS APPROPRIATE APPETITE

How do you make a fat rat? Give him a big bowl of rat chow but no room to run around. It seems animals eat more when they're active, but their appetites don't always shrink when they're inactive. According to several studies, the same is true for the "homo sedentarius" species, and it creates a problem. With the metabolic slowdown that accompanies inactivity, even a minimal food intake can foster a gain in body fat. This situation may explain why the secretary by day who watches sitcoms by night is constantly fighting with her fat: there may be a minimum activity threshold necessary for her "appestat" (appetite-regulating thermostat) to function properly.

Warning: if you find yourself in the paradoxical position of doing less but eating more these days, don't assume that cutting back on food (i.e., "dieting") is the key to the puzzle. Since appetite depends on activity, the logical solution is to do more; enjoy your RDA ("recommended daily activity") every day.

Living Lean students often report, "I'm not so hungry now that I've started walking," and there is some proof that activity aids appropriate appetite. As aerobic effort mobilizes fat for fuel, it shuts down hunger, at least for a while. But more interesting is what happens for the next couple of days.

Trial	Net Calorie Intake the Following Two Days
A. 60 minutes aerobic activity	2,900
B. 30 minutes aerobic activity	3,190
C. 30 minutes high- and low-intensity activity (1 minute anaerobic, 3 minutes aerobic)	3,980
D. No activity	3,230

In this West Virginia University experiment, untrained women who did a 60-minute treadmill workout (Trial A) not only burned the most calories, they also ate the least for two additional days. Thirty minutes was second best (Trial B), but combined high- and low-intensity effort (Trial C) actually increased food intake after incinerating the fewest calories—little gain for the pain.

Other reports similarly suggest that "killer" aerobics or start-and-stop sports like tennis are unpredictable when it comes to fat loss. Until it is understood why, be sure to enjoy some sustained, mid-level aerobic activity in addition to your favorite sports.

Later, after you have faithfully pounded the track or trail long enough, your newfound lean will start demanding extra calories and effortlessly burning them up. Runners constantly amaze their "jog-me-not" friends by outeating them—2,672 versus 1,970 calories in one comparison—while maintaining their lean advantage. Think how much fun you could have with an extra 700 calories every day—or even half that much! Aerobic activity might even change *what* you're hungry for. One exercise physiologist noted how his appetite for red meat, fatty foods, and sweets blossomed while he was sidelined from jogging due to an injury.

Few athletes or wild animals (or is that animals and wild athletes?) become overfat. But just confine them to buildings, cars, or cages—like our fat rats—and see what happens. Of course you may never achieve "elite athlete" status, and your training table might not ever sag under the weight of 3,000 well-earned calories. (Some athletes eat and burn as many as 10,000 calories a day!) But as you get in better shape, you'll find your appetite comes closer to matching your energy expenditure. *Super fitness means more food, less body fat.*

WHERE DO THE CALORIES GO?

Do you ever wonder where all your daily calories go? A big chunk of them, 75 percent, are needed just for maintenance operations—to keep your body heated, your heart beating, your lungs working, and your brain in gear. Another 15 percent (or more if you are quite active) are used to fuel physical activity. But the oddest and perhaps most important calorie drain is called "diet-induced

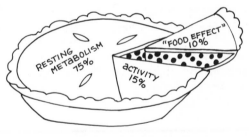

"Where Do the Calories Go?"

thermogenesis." Each time you eat, your metabolism (rate of calorie burning) increases. At the end of a day's eating, you may have disposed of up to 10 percent of your total calories.

To test this mysterious food effect, eight lean, muscular men were matched with eight overfat men of the same weight as well as the same height, age, and fitness level. From the outset, the lean men had the advantage of a faster resting metabolism (indicated by solid lines for both groups). After they drank a 750-calorie liquid meal, the lean men demonstrated an even greater advantage due to the food effect (broken lines for both groups). When compared with the overfat group, the lean group showed a 70 percent greater increase in metabolism while resting, a 310 percent greater increase while biking, and a 275 percent greater increase after biking (light versus dark shaded areas).

In other words, the lean guys burn off the food they eat better than the overfat guys, even while doing the exact same physical work—an almost unfair advantage. Their greater lean-to-fat ratio appears to be responsible for the difference, since both groups are the same weight.

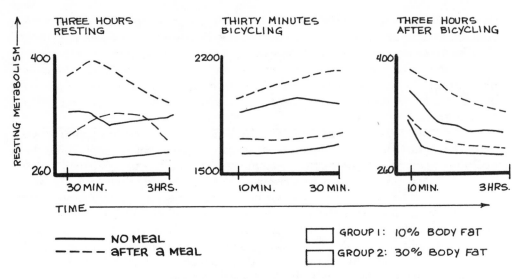

How Eating Boosts Metabolism

When you think about it, every piece of the metabolic pie is affected by how much lean you have (in proportion to fat) and how much you use it. And if eating and aerobic activity both burn extra calories, we should try to do both more often.

SOME LIKE IT HOT!

There's more to metabolism than meets the eye, and eating spicy foods evidently burns more than your palate. In one study, only a half teaspoon each of hot chili sauce and spicy mustard with a meal were able to boost metabolic rate 25 percent for several hours. So pour a pitcher of ice water to fight the fire; hot tamales, spicy gumbo, and pepper shrimp are the latest—and leanest—cuisine.

Fitness: Beyond Good Intentions

Do your health club dues make you feel guilty? Are your brand new jogging shoes gathering dust on the closet floor? Are you secretly glad the weather's so hot (cold, rainy) that no sane soul would expect you to venture outside? Even with the best of intentions, it's hard to stay on the fitness track and out of the recliner chair. But whatever your aerobic obstacles, concentrate on finding some way to get around them.

For women, safety is a constant concern. One woman who lives on a lonely country lane—and some city gals who must walk before or after work when it's dark—will pace up and down the block, only venturing as far as it seems safe. For more security, you might want to carry along dog repellent or mace; a shriek alarm (it can't be turned off once activated); or a beeper that's being monitored somewhere.

If you would really enjoy walking outdoors all the time but work schedules and the weather refuse to comply, perhaps you can track down a fitness facility where it's never too cold or too hot, where it never rains or snows, where it's never dangerously deserted, and where water, restrooms, and telephones are always close at hand. Where even a wheelchair athlete can make the rounds, and all the dogs have big button eyes, felt teeth, and pink ribbon collars. Sound like a Shangri-la? Not quite—that facility is the nearest shopping mall. Take a friend and your breakfast-to-go, and enjoy a first peek at the shoppers' specials as well as year-round fitness.

Nor should you have to cancel your aerobic obligations because of a physical impairment. Ask your physician to recommend a physical therapist who can set up a heart, lung, and muscle-strengthening program for you. One man who is recovering from surgery walks while holding on to a wheelchair for support. When he gets tired, he sits in it and works his arms. An elderly man fearful of straying too far from his house due to a heart condition now walks up and down his long driveway several times first thing in the morning. He returns to phone a neighbor at 8:00 A.M. on the dot to let her know all is well.

For the majority of us, however, aerobic obstacles are mental more than they are physical. Aerobic activity is not likely to happen if we just sit around and wait for it; in the modern world it must be intentional, and a little creativity helps.

For instance, one woman does calisthenics while she visits with a particularly grouchy shut-in, whenever she watches television, and during each phone call—fitness gossip, she calls it. Another woman bicycles while her teenage son jogs alongside. Since she has a one-speed bicycle, both of them enjoy an excellent workout.

Do any of these rationalizations sound familiar?

- "I know I should walk (jog, swim). I just don't do it." You're not alone. But why not become a member of the fitness in-crowd instead of the do-nothing bunch?
- "Because getting started is so difficult." Add "for anyone." The first day of spring training is never easy for a wintered-over football player, either. Simply take a walk break one day, then another day, and before you know it, getting started is history.
- "It's too strenuous." But easier than mowing and trimming the yard. And any athletic endeavor gets easier and easier with time.
- "It's dangerous." But not as deadly as being inactive. After a heart attack or surgery, the patient is rousted out of bed to walk as soon as possible—that's how important it is.
- "It's a chore." But surely more entertaining and uplifting than washing dishes or doing laundry.
- "It takes too long." Yet no longer than a half-hour TV show.
- "I don't have time." Could you squeeze extra minutes out of your lunch hour? Or put the potatoes in the oven or the stew in the pot and walk while they're cooking?
- "It's too dark when I get home." Invest in a stationary bicycle or head out to the gym. Or take an early-bird trek—you'll be hungry for breakfast when you get back and ready to tackle the day.
- "I don't work out because I'm too lazy." *Au contraire!* You are lazy because you don't work out. It's a fact: physical activity is an energy generator.
- "I can't stick with it." Moving more makes you *want* to move more; and if it's fun, it's addicting.
- "Some things are more important." But then, some things are less important. If you can figure out which ones they are, shove them aside occasionally. Is the compensation for a half hour of overtime as valuable as lean health? Does anyone really check to see whether your beds are made every day or the bathtub is spotless?

- "I'd work out if someone made me do it." That somebody is *you*, so pay your fee and join a fitness class. Park the bicycle where it's handy to grab. Leave your walking shoes by the door. Don't wait until you get trapped in a no-option situation.

That's exactly what happened to Marvin, an international business specialist with high blood pressure, high blood cholesterol, excess body fat, and chronic chest pains. "I never made a fitness commitment because for years I wasn't sure where I'd be at 5:30 every day. Now I realize I might not be anywhere at *any* hour of the day if I don't set some priorities."

 ## HURDLING AEROBIC OBSTACLES

List the reasons you haven't yet taken your first fitness walk, ride, or swim. Or catalogue some of the interferences that always keep you from your appointed aerobic rounds. Then wrestle each roadblock out of your way, one by one. Remember, nothing can stop you if you are determined nothing *can* stop you.

Aerobic Obstacles	How to Remove Them

A Walk a Day Keeps the Fat at Bay

BE AN ACTIVIST!

There are a few energy-savers you probably wouldn't want to do without—extension phones, floors that never need waxing, electric ice cream freezers (or better yet, ready-to-eat ice cream), dishwashers, washing machines, car washes, power steering, automatic sprinklers, and furnaces that supply a woodpile of heat at the flip of a switch.

Lest you write off the impact of these convenience gizmos, consider: a secretary who trades her manual typewriter for an electric model could gain 3 to 6 pounds (of fat) from calories saved in only a year's time. Just fighting the commuter traffic with a stick shift instead of an automatic transmission burns 33 percent more calories every day.

But most machines save minutes, too, so the bottom line is even more divergent: eight times more calories to shovel the snow than to blow it; seven times more calories to hang the laundry than to toss it in the dryer; and four times more calories to wash the dishes by hand. These savings quickly add up to costly fat-pounds. Perhaps you should inventory your appliances and the years you've owned each. Have they generated a void where physical activity used to be?

It's not necessary to go caveman in order to regain your lost health and fitness. But the establishment *is* weighted against moving. If someone offers you a ride, for instance, say, "No thanks, I enjoy the walk." You will doubtless evoke curious looks, even outright resistance (especially if you are dressed for success rather than dressed for recess). Your golf partners may be puzzled that you shun the cart; a tennis buddy may be amazed that you bike to the court rather than cruise up in your Maserati; your sunbathing friends may wonder why you wear yourself out swimming laps or walking the beach; the neighbors may think it odd that you navigate the neighborhood in the pouring rain, parasol and all. Let them puzzle, wonder, or stare. Once they get wind of the Big Benefits, you may find them begging to tag along.

Even if it's not branded "fitness," you can still reap heart-and-lung conditioning in the midst of the daily jungle. When a crowd is bottlenecked at the elevator, save time and head for the stairs. Avoid parking-space panic and add some diversion to your lunch hour by walking to and from the restaurant. On a long business trip, trade a coffee break for a walking break at a city park.

Chores and errands are inescapable, too, so why not make the most of them? You can congratulate yourself for getting the work done (it has to be done anyway), getting it done quickly, and providing some conditioning benefits at the same time. For example, a succession of short chores can be piggybacked: sweeping the garage, carrying the trash, energetically vacuuming the carpet, hauling laundry up and down the stairs, hanging it out to dry, tilling the garden. No doubt you can come up with a half hour's worth of chores begging for attention at your house every week.

One Living Lean student turned in her new-fashioned power mower for an old-fashioned push mower. Now she can mow early without disturbing the neighbors. A college student discovered that carrying groceries home from the store doubled the intensity of her walk. An attorney sacrificed a much-coveted parking space downtown to bike to work. And if your job, school, laundry, convenience store, newsstand, five-and-dime, post office, library, or park are within walking or biking distance, make a solemn vow you will no more resort to four wheels, wasted gas, and time lost looking for a parking spot. Be alert for any opportunities to get *out* of the driver's seat.

CHOOSE TO MOVE

When performed with vigor and enthusiasm, most any of these chores or recreational activities can be good calorie-burners. Add some music and an upbeat attitude, and you'll find work can be a lot like play.

Circle all activities you could do or would like to do.

Walking—the dog, with baby stroller, hiking, uphill, climbing, orienteering, treadmill, walking tours, outdoor festivals, nature walks, mall walking, parking lot perimeter, train station, walking track

Aerobics classes—high-impact, low-impact, TV program, videotape

Swimming, waterskiing, scuba diving, snorkeling

Snow skiing—cross country, downhill; snowshoeing, sledding

Canoeing, kayaking, rowing, using a rowing machine, rafting, river tubing, sailing, windsurfing

Cycling—outdoor, stationary

Jogging, running

Dancing—aerobic, jazz, disco, square, country-western, polka, clog, folk, ballroom, ballet

Roller skating, ice skating, hockey

Handball, racquetball

Tennis, badminton, volleyball, table tennis

Soccer, basketball, football, softball

Medicine ball, Frisbee, catch

Trampoline, mini-trampoline, gymnastics

Weight lifting, calisthenics, circuit training, jumping rope

Golf, bowling, fishing, primitive camping, horseback riding, hunting

Shuffleboard, horseshoes, pool and billiards

Showering, dressing

Folding and hanging laundry, changing beds, ironing, cooking, washing dishes, bathing the dog, picking up

Scrubbing, mopping, waxing, sweeping, vacuuming

Washing windows, cleaning pool, washing and waxing car

Carrying children—in baby carrier, in arms; playing with children

Shopping and running errands, delivering products, canvassing the neighborhood

Walking to work, walking to public transportation, using stairs

Yard work—raking leaves, mowing, trimming, watering, gardening

Carpentry, hammering, sawing, home repairs

Scraping and painting

Lifting, hauling, or moving furniture, boxes, or equipment, cleaning out garage

Digging, clearing brush, cutting firewood, chopping, working with a pick, farm chores

Shoveling sand, snow, dirt, ashes

 ## ACTIVITY LOG: A DAY IN THE LIFE

Why would someone make you sit, stand, or lie very still for all but a couple of hours out of a 24-hour day? Because you're a passenger on a nonstop flight around the world, or working as a live model in a department store window, or suffering cruel and unusual punishment at the federal pen? None of the above! No, you're just experiencing the average American's typically immobile day.

How about you? Is your backfield in motion enough of the time? There's one good way to find out. For each hour during an average day, check (✓) the activity level that best applies, as illustrated in the Sample Activity Log.

- Do you have at least two hours at the level of routine walking or better? (the last three columns)

- Do you have at least 30 minutes (preferably one hour) of brisk walking or better? (the last two columns)

Some things you can't change: giving up sleep *would* be cruel and unusual, and a desk job is a desk job. But you could stand while talking on the phone, or walk instead of catching a ride with a friend, or step briskly instead of dragging your feet. Cross the bridge from inertia to initiative!

Time	Sleep Lie, Sit	Stand	Routine Walking, Light Chores	Brisk Walking, Heavy Chores	Extreme Exertion	Notes
6 am to 8 am	✓	— —	✓ —	— —	— —	*getting ready for work*
8 am to 10 am	—✓—	— —	— —	— —	— —	*driving to work*
10 am to 12 pm	—✓—	— —	— —	— —	— —	*sitting at desk* — —
12 pm to 2pm	— —	✓ —	— —	— —	— —	*drive to lunch, sit and eat*
2 pm to 4 pm	—✓—		✓	— —	— —	*sitting at desk / walking*
4 pm to 6 pm	—✓—			— —	— —	*sit* — —
6 pm to 8 pm	— —	— —	✓	— —	— —	*jog (40 min) chores (20 min)*
8 pm to 10 pm	— —	— —	— —	— —	— —	— —
10 pm to 12 am	— —	— —	— —	— —	— —	— —

The Bridge

SMALL STEPS ADD UP

"I'm on my feet all day," complains the waitress whose swollen ankles echo her bulging waistline. "I supervise four construction sites," brags the superintendent with the health-threatening pot belly. "I get plenty of exercise around the house," says the mother of three who can't squeeze into her prepregnancy clothes. Although routine work burns calories, unless it's continuous and aerobic, it probably won't burn enough calories fast enough to reward you with noticeable fat reduction. On the other hand, 45 minutes a day of light to moderate activity like dancing, bowling, yard work, golf, or walking can reduce your risk of heart attack by one-third. And 3½ to 6½ total miles moved during the day can reduce that risk up to one-half.

You might want to pick up a pedometer at a sporting goods store and see how you measure up; overfat women average 3 miles in motion during a typical day while overfat men chalk up 6; lean women, on the other hand, put in around 7½ miles while lean men accrue 10. The final verdict seems to be this: if you're moving instead of sitting, you're building health, and health is Living Lean's priority goal.

✓ PRACTICE: SWING INTO ACTION

Can you find a way to make physical activity inescapable? If you have to cancel the car pool, buy recreational gear, or trade your electric appliances for hand-powered models, then do so.

Every day this week, see how much motion you can squeeze into your usual schedule—*in addition* to your aerobic workout. Look for clever "action ideas" that

ACTIVITY LOG

	Brisk Walking, Heavy Chores	Extreme Exertion	Notes

The Bridge

Time	Sleep Lie, Sit	Stand	Routine Walking, Light Chores
6 am to 8 am			
8 am to 10 am			
10 am to 12 pm			
12 pm to 2pm			
2 pm to 4 pm			
4 pm to 6 pm			
6 pm to 8 pm			
8 pm to 10 pm			
10 pm to 12 am			

can become permanent additions to your lifestyle, and log one or two suggestions on your Practice Diary. For instance, you could

- climb the stairs instead of taking the elevator
- do housework in time to polka music
- hand-saw a few logs for the fireplace
- go dancing on Fridays
- go bowling on Saturdays
- walk the dog after dinner

If you're female, don't forget to add some muscle work each day to give your bones the positive stress they need (see Strong Women).

You might even want to devise a contest with family members or co-workers. See who can come up with the best (fun, convenient) labor-*spending* ideas. Ingenuity wins the prize: every minute you aren't parked on the sofa means more bottom-line calories burned.

PRACTICE: PERSONAL TIME OUT

"I hope I haven't forgotten to thank anyone." If you have earned an Academy Award for your efforts toward Living Lean, don't overlook the principal character in the cast—you. Everybody needs to feel their hard work is appreciated, and you can't sit around waiting for acknowledgment from those in the wings—you might be waiting a long time!

Since you earned it, go ahead and take it: a 30-minute Personal Time Out, twice a day. Opt for a long coffee break or sit and soak in the tub. Curl up with a good detective story or daydream on the city bus. Take a picnic lunch break or skip out of a boring meeting. Some people enjoy aerobic activity so much it qualifies for time-out status, too.

Be advised that your Daily Prime Time is not goofing-off time. Put the "ought tos" in the closet for a half hour and haul out the "want tos." This is your chance to recharge and fill in the gaps; you not only deserve it, you need it. It has been said (and we hope it isn't so) that overeaters tend to everyone else's needs first, and their own needs last. Food is always a handy—though terribly uncreative—reward. Here's your chance to come up with some alternatives and prove the soothsayers wrong.

List below 15 things you like to do, then *do* them regularly.

Sticks and Stones and Sturdy Bones

If you fancy yourself trekking the Himalayas when you're 65 rather than reclining in an invalid's chair, don't wait until you book your passage to India to bolster your bone structure. If you are a young woman, it's not too soon—or, more correct, too late—to deposit some extra calcium in your bone "bank" so you will have access to it later in life.

If you are over 35 years old, you can still slow your bone mineral loss. If you don't make the effort, you may be minus as much as 25 percent of your bone mass by the time your Himalayan holiday rolls around. One of every *five* women suffers some kind of fracture due to osteoporosis, the brittle bone disease, by the time she turns 65; one of every *six* with hip fractures will die within a year. Those are not odds that inspire one to wager!

Calcium is your primary bone-boosting mineral, but it can't work all by itself. Magnesium, manganese, copper, zinc, boron, silicon, and vitamins A, C, D, and K are just a few skeleton-supporting nutrients. Chronic "dieting" is thus a liability: it's tricky enough to get adequate vitamins and minerals with an optimum calorie intake, and it's nearly impossible when you start skimping on food.

Too much protein, especially from meat, may also hasten bone loss; unfortunately, more than enough protein is par for the course in Western societies. On the other hand, vegetarians who use dairy products are in good shape nutritionally and great shape structurally. One study of lacto-vegetarians revealed 23 percent greater bone density at age 50 and 32 percent greater density at age 70 than was found in their meat-eating counterparts, even though calcium intakes were similar.

Perhaps you are already losing your height because your spine is shrinking, or you may have periodontal disease. Either condition places you in a high-risk category. Dr. Dee Jennings, a Dallas orthopedic surgeon, describes the typical fracture patient he wheels into surgery: "A slender, sedentary woman of northern European or Oriental descent who has a fair complexion, probably smokes cigarettes, and has breastfed several children; she has a dietary deficiency of calcium and vitamin D and gets little exercise or sunshine." Add a hysterectomy or menopause to the picture, and a very shaky bone structure crumbles completely apart.

One solution is to correct the nutritional deficit with Quality Control eating. Be especially stingy when treating yourself to the Spoilers caffeine and alcohol—they are notorious bone breakers. Sugar also drains body calcium, as do soft drinks with or *without* sugar (they pack too much phosphorus)..

You also need calcium on the table every day. Best choices are milk, yogurt, buttermilk, or cheese—preferably low-fat versions since fat inhibits calcium absorption. When dairy products are absent, legumes and other vegetables have to take up the calcium slack.

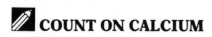 **COUNT ON CALCIUM**

Using the Calcium Counter, determine your typical daily calcium intake. Be sure to consider your usual serving size for each item.

Calcium Counter

Yogurt, plain low-fat	1 cup	415* mg
Milk	1 cup	300
Sardines, with bones	2 ounces	247
Natural cheese	1 ounce	195

Shrimp	2 ounces	182
Processed cheese	1 ounce	169
Salmon, with bones	2 ounces	111
Broccoli, turnip or beet greens, okra, bok choy	½ cup	80–100
Navy, Great Northern, pinto, or garbanzo beans, cooked	1 cup	85
Tofu	3 ounces	80

Additional calcium sources ranging from 60 to 40 milligrams per serving: black-eyed peas, mustard greens, spinach, figs, oranges, almonds, Parmesan cheese, winter squash, corn tortillas, Brazil nuts, filberts, sesame and sunflower seeds.

*Commercial fruit-sweetened yogurt may have 70 milligrams less calcium.

Daily Calcium Intake

	Calcium (mg)
Milk, yogurt, buttermilk	_____
Cheese	_____
Legumes	_____
Vegetables	_____
Other	_____
Total	_____

Did you chalk up 800 milligrams, the current RDA? (A number of authorities believe 1,000 milligrams is a better goal for adults.) After menopause, women may need as much as 1,500 milligrams of calcium, plus additional estrogen, to fully protect their bones. It has been determined that our Paleolithic ancestors hunted and gathered at least 1,500 milligrams of calcium a day, so we must be somewhere in the right ball park.

If your good calcium-eating intentions fail, you may be in the market for a supplement. Calcium carbonate (or oyster shell) is probably the cheapest, but calcium citrate may be better absorbed, especially if you take it before or with a protein-containing meal. It doesn't seem to cause bloating or kidney stones, either. If plain calcium tablets aggravate constipation, consider using a brand that contains magnesium as well. Because of possible nutrient interactions, a multimineral with copper, zinc, and manganese may also be good insurance.

Don't forget a little fun in the sun, since you do need vitamin D to properly absorb calcium. If window glass, sunscreens, clothing, rain, or smog filter out too much ultraviolet light, you can turn to fortified milk, one of the few food sources of vitamin D. And although a good diet is essential, don't ignore the lifestyle risk factors you can correct. Otherwise, your bones will still come out on the losing end.

MAKING THE MOST OF MILK

"*I don't like milk.*" If you can't stomach the thought of drinking a glass of milk straight up, consider hiding it in foods like soups, puddings, pancakes, or hot cereals prepared with milk instead of water. Earn more calcium at breakfast by spiking your cereal milk with a spoonful of nonfat dry milk. The same trick works for baked products or casseroles—you'll never know it's there. Have you tried fruit with yogurt yet? You might like it. If you are a sour cream lover, try switching to yogurt or buttermilk as a base for salad dressing or as a sauce for veggies and baked potatoes.

"Milk doesn't like me." At least that's the way it seems, if you suffer diarrhea, gas, or bloating each time you attempt to drink your moo juice. People who can't digest the lactose in a big glass of milk will often do okay with a small cup of milk. Others must adopt low-lactose alternatives like yogurt, cheese, or cottage cheese. There is a special reduced-lactose milk for people with fussy intestines. Also look for Lactaid, a powdered enzyme you add to regular milk to cancel the lactose. Be aware that northern Europeans usually can digest lactose, but most of the world's people cannot. Your ethnic heritage helps determine which category you fall into.

DAIRY DELITES

With 400 milligrams of calcium, this tasty blender drink will help you wake up to half your daily calcium quota.

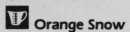 Orange Snow

1 cup skim milk
2 tablespoons nonfat dry milk
3 tablespoons frozen orange juice concentrate
3/4 teaspoon vanilla
Whirl all ingredients briefly in a blender.
1 recipe = 1 Fruit, 1 1/2 Milk

Eggnog Custard

This custard has a delicious aroma while baking, and it supplies 500 milligrams of calcium to boot.

1 cup skim or 1/2% milk	1/2 teaspoon vanilla
4 tablespoons nonfat dry milk	2 to 3 teaspoons honey
1 egg	sprinkle nutmeg
1 tablespoon rum	

Blend dry milk into liquid milk. Add egg and beat slightly. Stir in rum, vanilla, and honey; pour into large custard cup. Bake at 300 degrees for 30 to 35 minutes, or until firm.

1 recipe = 1 Protein, 1 Fruit (honey), 2 Milk

STRONG WOMEN

The Missing Link for many Western women is positive bone stress—as for muscles, it's use 'em or lose 'em. Weight-bearing sports like walking and jogging protect bone structure better than swimming or bicycling, but don't overlook the obvious. "No, dear, that's too heavy. Let me get it for you." Chivalry may be alive and well, but strong women are fast becoming an endangered species.

It may be unladylike to do manual work, but it's even less graceful to hobble around in a cast using a cane—the wages of too little calcium and not enough physical labor. If you should be able to but can't lift a spare tire out of the trunk, open a heavy office building door, or hoist a sack of dog food up the stairs, it's time to do as Scarlett O'Hara did and get physical. Welcome any opportunity to haul in the groceries, put the heavy boxes on the top shelf, or pick up a fussy toddler one more time. Remember the rule, though: breathe out as you lift, using your hips and bent knees; and keep your back straight.

If household chores don't exactly thrill you, put on a favorite record and do some calisthenics while grasping a couple of dumbbells, books, or sacks of dried beans. You might consider purchasing an old-fashioned medicine ball

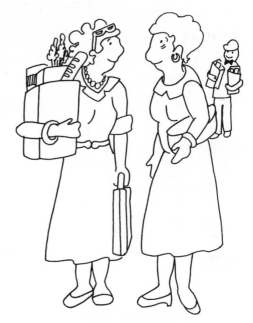

**Stress Your Bones
and Save Them from Destruction**

and drafting the whole family into some fun and games. Though it looks big and clumsy, the ball is soft and fairly light weight. Whatever your bone-building technique, you'll find physical strength gives you a feeling of psychological power, a confidence that says without reservation, "I can *do* it."

✐✓ Practice Diary Five

If the fitness message didn't hit home in Chapter 3, the preceding introduction to metabolism should convince you. As opposed to temporary "diets" that effect only superficial changes in your body, building lean and burning fat with aerobic activity stacks the deck so that it's easier for you to stay lean—permanently.

The fringe benefits from as little as two active hours a week are mighty impressive; and besides, being fit is the way you were meant to be—it's a natural. Living Lean *is* living fit.

RECORD MEALS AND SNACKS

SUNDAY

MONDAY

TUESDAY

WEDNESDAY

THURSDAY

FRIDAY

SATURDAY

LIVING LEAN

PRACTICE DIARY FIVE

Practices

Practices	Su	M	Tu	W	Th	F	Sa	Notes
Aerobic Activity—30 minutes, 4 days a week								
Record Meals and Snacks								
Swing into Action								
Personal Time Out—30 minutes, twice a day								

Day

✓ = yes, I did try;   ✓✓ = yes, I did well

Suggested Practices

- List aerobic obstacles and possible solutions in Hurdling Aerobic Obstacles.
- Keep an Activity Log for one to three days.
- Small Steps Add Up: buy a pedometer and determine the total miles you walk in a day; then try to increase that number.
- Try a new sport or activity from Choose to Move.
- Using the Calcuim Counter, calculate your average daily calcium intake; add food to meet the calcium RDA.

GOOD FOOD GUIDE TALLY

	Gr/St	Pro	Veg	Fruit	Milk	F/HF	Extras
Sug. Daily Por.							

Sug. Daily Por. Minimum = Suggested Daily Portions
Gr/St = Grain/Starch   Veg = Vegetables
Pro = Protein   F/HF = Fat/Hidden Fat

WEEK SIX

*Quantity Control Assurance
　　The Calorie Challenge: Adequate But Not Excessive

The Training Table: Practice Eating to Make Perfect
　　Pick a Plan, Set the Table
　　Modify Your Plan with Trade-Offs and Substitutions
　*Design a Menu
　　Practice: Plan/Record Meals and Snacks
　　Training Table Menus
　　Practice: Leave One Bite
　　Practice: Repeat Practice

*Practice Diary Six

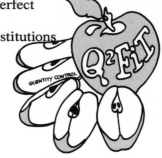

Quantity Control Assurance

Although packaged in an infinite variety of formats, the heart of most weight-loss "diets" is cutting down on calories. But is eating too much the primary source of your excess fat? Oddly, a lot of people decide they must cut calories even though they haven't the slightest idea how many calories they are supposed to eat, nor how many calories they *do* eat and thus whether they need to cut calories at all.

Try your hand at the following questions:

- How many calories do you eat (on an average day when you are not following a "diet" plan)? _____
- What is the calorie recommendation for a man or woman your age? _____

Read on, because the answers are all here.

"How many calories do you eat?" Using a calorie counter or the Good Food Guide for a rough estimate, accurately and honestly determine your calorie intake for three or more consecutive days, doing and eating as usual. Add the totals together and divide by the number of days to get an average. If your body weight and composition remain the same during this time, you are in calorie balance: the calories you eat match the calories you burn up.

Your current calorie intake (and expenditure): _____

"What is the calorie recommendation for a man or woman your age?" Your intake should fall somewhere in the range for your age group shown below, unless you are quite small, extremely inactive, or your metabolism has declined from frequent dieting. This recommended calorie intake is indirectly a recommendation for energy expenditure: an adult woman should be active enough to eat and burn 2,000 calories a day; an adult man, 2,700. Use the table below to find your recommended energy allowance (REA).

RECOMMENDED ENERGY ALLOWANCE*

Age	Calorie Recommendation	Recommended Calorie Range
Women		
19–22	2,100	1,700–2,500
23–50	2,000	1,600–2,400
51–75	1,800	1,400**–2,200
76 and up	1,600	1,200**–2,000
Men		
19–22	2,900	2,500–3,300
23–50	2,700	2,300–3,100
51–75	2,400	2,000–2,800
76 and up	2,050	1,650–2,450

*Based on a light activity level.

**It is very difficult to get adequate vitamins and minerals from foods when calories fall below 1,500 per day.

Source: Recommended Dietary Allowances, 9th ed. (Washington, D.C.: National Academy of Sciences, 1980).

Your calorie recommendation (REA): _____

If you would prefer a more individualized recommendation, you can use the technique introduced in Chapter 4. The additional calculations give you a more accurate number.

1. For men: write down 106.
   For women: write down 100.

   1. _____

2. For men: add 6 for each inch in height above 5 feet.
   For women: add 5 for each inch in height above 5 feet.

   2. _120_

3. Now wrap your thumb and middle finger around your wrist where it joins your hand.
   - If your fingers overlap, subtract 10 percent from the number in Step 2.
   - If your fingers meet, step 3 is the same as 2.
   - If there is a gap between your fingertips, add 10 percent to the number in step 2. Your calculated weight for height is the number in step 3. (This number is for calculating purposes only and should not be confused with so-called "ideal" weight.)

   3. _120_
   Weight for height

   $$\begin{array}{r} 120 \\ \times 15 \\ \hline 600 \\ 1200 \\ \hline 1800 \end{array}$$

4. Last, multiply the number in step 3 by one of the numbers in the left-hand column below. (If your activity varies from day to day, either take an average or create a range by using two calculations for two different activity levels.) Your suggested calorie intake, based on your size and activity, is the number in step 4.

   4. _____
   Suggested
   calorie intake

Multiply by:	If this is your activity level:
13	Inactive (Desk job with no activity or mostly sitting, such as a clerk. No regular organized activity during leisure time or less than once a week.)
15	Light Activity (On your feet part of the day, such as a teacher. Sporadic recreation—weekend golf or tennis; an occasional jog, swim, or bike ride; or walk three to four times a week.)

| 17 | Moderate Activity (Move or lift items, climb stairs, or engage in physical work at least half the day. Jog, swim, or cycle four to six times a week for 30 to 60 minutes, or walk four to six times a week for 60 minutes.) |
| 20+ | Very Active (Heavy labor most of the day, such as a roofer. Active sports five to six times a week for 60 minutes or more, or recreational or competitive athlete.) |

When you are estimating your activity, be sure to look at the whole day: are you basically a chair-sitter most of the time who jogs a half hour four times a week? The Activity Log in Chapter 5 may help you decide.

THE CALORIE CHALLENGE: ADEQUATE BUT NOT EXCESSIVE

It's nice to know how many calories you eat and how many calories healthy adults are supposed to eat. But your goal is to trim unwanted body fat. How many calories are right for that job? For a moderately overfat person, the answer is a challenge to the heart of the Living Lean philosophy: the *most* you can eat while continuing to burn body fat and preserving or building lean muscle.

Of course, most Living Lean students are eager to lose excess fat as fast as possible, but the fast way is not necessarily the best way. Your long-term health is a priority goal with Living Lean, and to protect it, you should lose *no more* than 10 to 15 percent of your body weight over any 9- to 18-month period.

Be careful *how* you accomplish this. When you cut calories without adding sufficient aerobic activity, you have adopted a "diet" in disguise. You risk both a slowing of your metabolism and the loss of lean tissue. (If you are moderately overfat, you probably can't afford to give up much—if any—of your lean. Very heavy people may have added extra muscle to support their extra fat. *That* lean is expendable.)

Luckily, aerobic activity can prevent lean loss associated with "dieting," but it doesn't work every time. (In one 1,250-calorie diet study, for example, 30 minutes of aerobic activity six days a week produced weight loss that was only 70 percent fat—the rest was lean.) Plus most successful studies have included fairly vigorous, supervised exercise. If there's a chance your aerobic intentions may get preempted some days, you would be wise to cut calories with utmost caution, if at all. Fitness comes *first*, food intake must *follow*.

So we're back to the question: how many calories are right for the job at hand? To best pull body fat out of storage, you need enough calories, but then not too many. Instead of restricting calories first and then working your way up to a maintenance level (a process that may incur a metabolic and psychological penalty), Living Lean takes a different approach: start right where you are now, and then adjust toward an optimum calorie level for health.

If your calorie intake is already below the recommended range for your age, don't restrict further unless you are a very tiny person. Instead, stick with that amount and switch your focus to physical activity, so you can gradually *increase* your calories to a nutritionally adequate level.

Otherwise, begin with your current or recommended calorie intake (whichever is less), and then decrease only slightly *if necessary*. A small reduction—say, 250 calories a day, or 10 to 15 percent less than your usual intake—will better protect your lean and be less likely to trigger a decline in metabolic rate. Reread Chapters 4 and 5 (the effect of "diets" on metabolism and nutrition) before making a more drastic reduction.

As noted in Chapter 2, it is possible for you to lose fat even *without* a deliberate calorie restriction, so long as you (1) increase your aerobic activity and (2) choose most of your foods from the Good Food Guide—especially those high in fiber and low in fat.

When you decide on an optimum calorie level to continue your Living Lean project, fill in that number here: _____.

The Training Table:
Practice Eating to Make Perfect

You may snicker when someone suggests you need to "practice" eating. But there's a right way and a wrong way for everything—including how, what, when, where, and why you eat. The right kind of practice will generate better eating habits.

Athletes figure eating at the training table will improve their performance. Now that you are in training, you can look forward to your Training Table, too. Lest there be any mistake, this is not a "diet." It is rather an eat-and-learn experience: you try out some nutritious, balanced menus for a couple of days (or weeks) and observe your physical and psychological response.

Since your goal is to become a reeducated eater, try not to put your brain on automatic pilot when you're experimenting with a new food or combination. Instead, ask yourself questions about the experience. Do you look forward to eating this food again? Does it look good on your plate? Does it taste good? Is it filling and psychologically satisfying? Could you learn to prepare this food? Can you find some version of it at a restaurant? If the menus aren't appropriate for you, can you adapt them so they are?

If you are accustomed to gorging yourself when you sit down to a meal, examine how it feels to undereat for a change. Tell yourself it's okay not to feel stuffed when the meal is finished, and promise yourself a piece of fresh fruit for dessert an hour or two after dinner.

If you are used to eating very little or nothing at all until dinnertime, gradually introduce some foods early in the day. You may feel more comfortable with small, equal-sized meals, plus snacks to fill the hungry gaps in between. Remember, high-fiber foods are filling but not fattening, and you need the vitamins and minerals they provide to get and stay lean and healthy.

If you've put in extra hours of work or play, instead of grabbing a double helping of ice cream or pastry, opt for a higher-calorie Training Table to satisfy your surplus appetite. If you indulge in a banquet-sized meal late one evening, you might select a lighter Training Table the next day or two. (Your body should perform this balancing act automatically—watch and see if it does.)

Since the Training Table is just what it claims—elementary education for eating lean—sooner or later you will graduate to find your own appetite planning and selecting healthful meals for you, without the necessity of cheat sheets (printed menus). But whenever you need a refresher course, the Training Table will be standing by—whether one day a week or one week a month—to jog your memory.

PICK A PLAN, SET THE TABLE

You have three options for setting your Training Table. The easiest is to choose foods primarily from the Good Food Guide in Chapter 4, paying attention to the suggested minimum daily servings from each food group to ensure good nutrition.

If you'd like to keep closer tabs on your calorie intake, try the second option: choose one of the Portion Plans listed in the chart below, based on your proposed optimum calorie intake from the Calorie Challenge. Each plan tells you how many portions to eat from each food group per day. Then you can use the Good Food Guide to help you select specific foods and amounts.

Next to each plan there is an alternate plan listed in brackets. It has the same number of calories but a greater percentage of carbohydrate; thus, it's a little more challenging for the meat and cheese lover. You can also add or subtract food portions to make your plan fit any desired calorie level. (For instance, you may prefer to eat 1,500 calories instead of 1,650.) Just use the Quick Calorie Check to verify your total calories.

Although there are separate plans designated for women and for men, a man can use the 2,000-calorie plan and a woman can use the 1,800-calorie plan, for example. Keep in mind that 1,350 calories (for women) and 1,800 calories (for men) are pretty much rock-bottom recommendations. The 1,650- and 2,300-calorie plans match the usual calorie intake for adults, while the 2,000 and 2,700 plans satisfy the adult RDA for calories. The Max Plan is suitable only for a very lean or very active adult. Be sure to double the portion size for Grain/Starch and Fruit.

Regardless of your choice, the fat calories for *all* plans equal less than 30 percent of total calories, as recommended by the U.S. Dietary Goals. Should you opt for proteins primarily from the Lean Protein List (see Chapter 4) and use mostly skim milk or yogurt, then your fat intake will be closer to 25 percent of calories or less.

On the other hand, if you eat out a lot, buy processed products, and indulge often in foods from the Fat and Hidden Fat lists (see Chapter 4), your fat calories could exceed a healthy range. If this sounds like your lifestyle, you might want to substitute reduced-calorie versions of margarine, mayonnaise, and salad dressing whenever possible or eliminate one or two of the suggested Fat portions each day.

✏️ QUICK CALORIE CHECK

To double-check how many calories you are eating, just multiply the number of portions by the calories per portion.

Number of Portions		Calories per Portion		Calories
Grain/Starch _5 _16_	×	80 _560_ _480_	=	_400_
Protein _3_	×	75 _225_	=	_225_
Vegetable _4_	×	25 _100_	=	_100_
Fruit _4_	×	60 _180_	=	_240_
Milk (skim) _1_	×	90 _90_	=	_90_
(low-fat) _____	×	120 _²135_	=	_____
Fat _3_	×	45 _290_	=	_135_
		Total Calories		_1185_

Select one of the following plans with an appropriate calorie level for you. Fill in this "Suggested Daily Portions" on the Good Food Guide Tally in Practice Diary Four. This is now your *recommended* daily intake for each food group instead of a suggested minimum.

Portion Plans for Women*

Food Group	1,350 Calories**		1,650 Calories		2,000 Calories		3,000 to 3,450 Calories‡
Grain/Starch	5	7	7	9	9	11	7–8 (double portions)
Protein	5	3	6	4	7	5	7–9
Vegetable†	3+	3+	4+	4+	5+	5+	5–7+
Fruit	3	3	3½	3½	4	4	5 (double portions)
Milk	2	2	2	2	2	2	2–3
Fat	3	4	3	4	5	5	10

Portion Plans for Men*

Food Group	1,800 Calories		2,300 Calories		2,700 Calories		3,000 to 3,450 Calories‡
Grain/Starch	8	9	10	11	12	13	7–8 (double portions)
Protein	7	4	8	5	9	6	7–9
Vegetable†	3+	4+	5+	5+	7+	7+	5–7+
Fruit	3	4	4	5	5	6	5 (double portions)
Milk	2	2	2½	2½	3	3	2–3
Fat	5	6	6	8	7	9	10

*An alternate plan, higher in carbohydrate, is listed in brackets for each calorie level.

**It is very difficult to get adequate vitamins and minerals from foods when calories fall below 1,500 per day.

†Vegetables are ad-lib foods. The numbers listed are minimums, not maximums.

‡Max Plan for active men and women.

SAMPLE GOOD FOOD GUIDE TALLIES

1650 calories   **ONE-DAY RECORD**

Sug. Daily Por.	Gr/St	Pro	Veg	Fruit	Milk	F/HF	Extras
	7	63	4+	3½	2	3	
B	2			2	1	1	
S							sugar doughnut
L	2	4				2	
S							2 small cookies
D	1	3	3			4	
S				1			
Total	5	7	3	3	1	7	✓✓

Sug. Daily Por. = Suggested Daily Portions
Gr/St = Grain/Starch   Veg = Vegetables
Pro = Protein   F/HF = Fat/Hidden Fat

**2000 calories
[high-carbo plan]**   **SEVEN-DAY RECORD**

Sug. Daily Por.	Gr/St	Pro	Veg	Fruit	Milk	F/HF	Extras
	11	5	5+	4	2	& 5	
	₪₪	₪ I	////	///	//	₪ //	I
	₪ I	₪ ///	///	₪	I	₪I	

Sug. Daily Por. = Suggested Daily Portions
Gr/St = Grain/Starch   Veg = Vegetables
Pro = Protein   F/HF = Fat/Hidden Fat

One woman in the Living Lean program first decided to use the 1,650-calorie plan. However, extra candy, ice cream, and pastry didn't fade out of her eating life until she switched to the 1,800-calorie, high-carbohydrate plan; 1,650 calories simply weren't enough for her, as evidenced by the circled totals on the two Sample Good Food Guide Tallies on page 115 and above. The 2,000-calorie high-carbohydrate plan was selected by a man who eats out often, so he allows himself one less Fat portion each day to accommodate fat hidden in his restaurant meals. Even so, he needs to account for as much of the fat he eats as possible.

If your taste buds are happy without lots of margarine, gravy, or salad dressing, don't retrain them just to fill your Fat quota for the day. And if you don't regularly prepare your own meals, use fat-skimmed ingredients or read labels carefully; it's better to come up short—not long—on total Fat portions. At more than 100 calories per tablespoon, unrecognized fat can really undermine your meal-planning efforts.

MODIFY YOUR PLAN WITH TRADE-OFFS AND SUBSTITUTIONS

A healthy appetite is a good sign, but constant, unsatisfied hunger spells big trouble. You should *not* be hungry while using the Training Table. If you are, switch to a higher-calorie plan or menu, or reach for extra carbohydrate and fiber foods from the triangle on the left in the diagram below. Be cautious about adding fiberless foods from the triangle on the right; they may shove you over your Protein or Fat limit for the day.

More often it's the Extras that grab your appetite, and whether or not you are aware of it, they displace calories from other, more nutritious sources. So think twice before giving up a nutritious food in exchange for sweets, alcohol, or fatty or fried foods. As stated before, Fat portions are the logical trade for Extras, but there are only so many available for trade.

You *can* afford occasional switches within or between triangles to accommodate your changing needs. In the heat of summer, you might crave light fruit or pasta salads instead of cooked vegetables or heavy proteins. And on a frostbitten February day, you might be more tempted by a hearty vegetable stew with meat or bean protein than by chilly fruits and juices. It's like a TV game show in some ways; you can buy some extra Protein portions (such as 6 ounces of barbecued chicken at a picnic), but in exchange you should sell (bypass) the big dollop of butter on your bread. This is *your* project; do it however it works best for you.

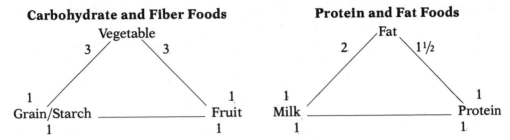

Carbohydrate and Fiber Foods	Protein and Fat Foods

The sides of these triangles connect calorie equivalents. Here's an example of a triangle trade: if you give up 1 Fruit portion, you could add 3 extra Vegetable portions for about the same calories.

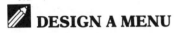 **DESIGN A MENU**

After figuring out what and how much to eat, some Living Lean students still want to know what foods to eat at which meals. The answer is, it doesn't matter so long as you end up with close to the right portion totals at the end of the day.

To help you plan a whole day's eating, you can use the Sample Menu Design chart. You'll notice Fruits are reserved for snacks, and Protein foods are distributed throughout the day instead of congregating at dinner. But these ideas—including the suggested number of Good Food Guide portions for each meal and snack—are just proposals. You might choose a lighter breakfast by switching morning Protein and Fat portions to later in the day; or you may prefer to serve Fruit portions with meals as dessert.

If your total portions for each food group match your Portion Plan, then you've developed a good, workable menu. Post it behind a kitchen cupboard door and refer to it daily.

SAMPLE MENU DESIGN

	Suggested Portion Number	Food Group	Good Food Guide Choices
	2–3	Grain/Starch	Cereal, bread, or muffin
	1	Protein	Egg, cheese, cottage cheese, or meat
BREAKFAST	1–2	Fruit	Fruit or juice
	1	Milk	Milk or yogurt
	1	Fat	Nuts, seeds, or margarine
	2–3	Grain/Starch	Bread or crackers
	1–2	Protein	Dried beans, cheese, or meat
LUNCH	1–3+*	Vegetable	Salad or vegetable
	1–2	Fat	Salad dressing
	2–3	Grain/Starch	Bread or rice and starchy vegetable
	1–3	Protein	Meat, cheese, or dried beans
DINNER	2–4+*	Vegetable	Salad and vegetables
	1–2	Fat	Salad dressing or margarine

SNACKS	1–2	Grain/Starch	Crackers or muffin
	1–3	Fruit	Fruit
	1	Milk	Milk or yogurt
	1–3	Fat	Nuts or seeds

*Vegetables are ad-lib foods. The numbers listed are minimums, not maximums.

Here's an example of a lunch and snack planned by using the Sample Menu Design:

	Portion Number	Food Group	Good Food Guide Choices
LUNCH	2	Grain/Starch	Turkey (1 ounce)
	1	Protein	Rye bread (2 slices)
	1	Vegetable	Garden salad (1 cup)
	2	Fat	Margarine (1 teaspoon) and Italian salad dressing (1 tablespoon)
SNACK	1	Fruit	Peach (1)
	1	Milk	Yogurt (1 cup)
	1	Fat	Almonds (6)

Now create one or several appetizing menus for yourself on the Sample Menu. Use your Portion Plan and the Sample Menu Design, and try them out. You don't have to use all the different food groups suggested for each meal. Just pick the ones you want and leave the others blank.

SAMPLE MENU

	Gr/St	Pro	Veg	Fruit	Milk	F/HF
Your Portion Plan						

	Portion Number	Food Group	Good Food Guide Choices
BREAKFAST	_____	Grain/Starch	
	_____	Protein	
	_____	Fruit	
	_____	Milk	
	_____	Fat	
SNACK	_____		
	_____		
LUNCH	_____	Grain/Starch	
	_____	Protein	
	_____	Vegetable	
	_____	Fruit	
	_____	Milk	
	_____	Fat	

SNACK $\left\{\begin{array}{l} \underline{\hspace{3em}} \\ \underline{\hspace{3em}} \\ \underline{\hspace{3em}} \end{array}\right.$

$\left\{\begin{array}{ll} \underline{\hspace{2em}} & \text{Grain/Starch} \\ \underline{\hspace{2em}} & \text{Protein} \\ \underline{\hspace{2em}} & \text{Vegetable} \\ \underline{\hspace{2em}} & \text{Fruit} \\ \underline{\hspace{2em}} & \text{Milk} \\ \underline{\hspace{2em}} & \text{Fat} \end{array}\right.$

SNACK $\left\{ \underline{\hspace{3em}} \right.$

FREE TO CHOOSE

"Just give me some menus with all the foods I'm supposed to eat so I don't have to think about it." Some clinics even sell preselected, premeasured foods for your eating convenience: no shopping, no cooking, and especially no decisions.

The problem with this too-good-to-be-true technique is that it's too good to be true. Recent evidence shows that "no choice" programs leave you without the tools to *make* choices, which you ultimately must do in a world where you can't escape the battle of the brands. People who request no-think techniques may not be ready to tackle genuine changes in lifestyle.

But you can fight for your right to choose. Refuse to let the "we'll do it for you" reducing schemes push you around any longer. Get off the "diet" merry-go-round, and start making some real headway on the road to Living Lean.

✅ PRACTICE: PLAN/RECORD MEALS AND SNACKS

Although it's fun to take potluck for meals and snacks occasionally, it can make your Living Lean project fairly hit or miss—and too often the latter. Luckily, there are a couple of easy ways to sharpen your aim:

- **Plan.** Write your proposed menus on your Practice Diary a day (or better, several days) in advance. Don't forget any important "details"—like shopping ahead for all those foods you plan to eat!
- **Record.** Jot down what you eat, as you eat it, on your Practice Diary—whether or not you *planned* ahead to eat it. Or carry a little notebook or card in your pocket for the same purpose.

When planning, use your Portion Plan to fill in the "Suggested Daily Portions" on your Good Food Guide Tally. Then compare the number of portions you'd like to eat with the number you actually eat. Where are the discrepancies? Since the emphasis this week is on Quantity Control, circle any total that *exceeds* the recommendation. (Remember that vegetables are ad-lib foods.) Write yourself a reminder about the food groups that are over or under your target so you can adjust your eating. And whenever you plan or record your meals and snacks, give yourself a check mark (✓/✓) for either or both accomplishments.

TRAINING TABLE MENUS

The third option for your Training Table is the following collection of high-fiber, low-fat, ready-made menus. A one-week sampler is included for each of three calorie levels: 1,350, 1,650, and 2,000 calories. A one-day sample is provided for 2,300 and 2,700 calories. Choose the level most appropriate for you.

Please note: these menus are neither totally idealistic nor totally realistic; rather, they rank somewhere in between. For example, beer, light desserts, and fast food (pizza) make an occasional guest appearance, while caffeine has taken a permanent vacation (the substitutes are so easy, and just as tasty). You'll notice also that meat turns up at most once a day, and some days not at all.

To get enough of some hard-to-come-by trace minerals, however, you need to eat either more meat (and thus more protein, cholesterol, and fat) than is healthy or more legumes than you may be willing (or perhaps able) to eat. Or you need to be active enough to eat and burn at least 2,500 to 3,000 calories a day, since more calories deliver more nutrients. Unless (or until) you fit that description, a nutritional supplement may be good insurance—especially if your accustomed eating style includes an occasional drink or dessert or if you eat fried, processed, or restaurant-prepared foods from time to time.

You can extract maximum nutrition from the presented menus by choosing real whole grain products and mixes as called for (Chapter 2 gives pointers on tracking down whole grains). Use primarily fresh or occasionally frozen fruits and vegetables. Steam or microwave veggies to retain important nutrients. Add small amounts of blackstrap molasses to boost iron, and brewer's yeast for extra B vitamins, particularly folacin. Remember that Vitamin C will increase the absorption of iron from your meal. And don't pass over dark-meat poultry; though somewhat higher in fat, it contains more iron and zinc than does the light meat.

To keep fat within 20 to 25 percent of total calories, use skim or ½ percent milk and plain (unsweetened) low-fat or nonfat yogurt. When the menu doesn't include added sugar or fat, try artificial sweetener, nonstick pan spray for cooking, butter-flavored granules, or no-oil salad dressing. Or stretch regular dressing by thinning it with yogurt, buttermilk, lemon juice, tomato juice, or vinegar. Use a margarine with liquid vegetable oil like safflower, corn, or soybean oil (a good source of vitamin E) listed first, and add just before eating to get more flavor from a smaller portion. Another suggestion: low-fat cheese tastes better served warm or at room temperature. And for any prepared product—from whole grain crackers to bottled tomato sauce—buy the brand with the least hidden fat and salt.

Approximate Good Food Guide portions are given for each food. Use them to help you change the menus to fit your tastes. If you don't care for bagels, for example, select a substitute Grain/Starch portion from the Good Food Guide. If you aren't crazy about chopped nuts on your breakfast flakes, save the Fat portion for margarine to fry your egg or spread on your toast. If suggested meals seem too large, divide them into smaller meals with extra snacks (eating more often is a good practice). If a big dinner invariably means you crave a big dessert, switch your main meal to lunch. What you need are new, workable ideas, and you should be able to find at least a few good ones here!

Training Table Menus

In the Training Table Menus, nutritional calculations were computed with N-Squared Computing software; daily calorie averages are within 30 calories of the categories listed. When there is a choice of menu items, the first item is used for calculations. The Good Food Guide portions listed are approximate only; except for Milk, there is no listing for less than ½ portion. A combined listing is used to identify hidden fat in baked goods like corn bread (e.g., 1 Grain/Starch-1 Fat portion) and nuts (e.g., 1 Protein-1 Fat portion per two tablespoons nuts); and also for one-half cup or more cooked dried beans (e.g., 1 Grain/Starch-½ Protein portion per one-half cup beans). Recipes found elsewhere in this book are in bold type.

1,350—DAY 1

Breakfast

1 cup old-fashioned oatmeal, 3 tablespoons blueberries or 1 to 2 teaspoons light maple syrup, 6 pecan halves	2 Grain/Starch 1½ Fat
1 cup skim milk, ½ cup orange juice	1 Milk, 1 Fruit

Lunch

Turkey taco: 1 whole wheat tortilla, 2 ounces diced light and dark turkey, ⅔ cup shredded leaf lettuce, ½ cup chopped tomato, 2 tablespoons chopped pumpkin seeds, 2 tablespoons sliced avocado, taco sauce, cumin, garlic, chili powder	1 Grain/Starch 2 Protein 1 Vegetable 1 Protein-1 Fat 1 Fat
6 ounces low-sodium V-8 vegetable juice	1½ Vegetable

Snack

Picante dip: ½ cup thick low-fat yogurt or buttermilk, spiced with 1 to 2 teaspoons hot salsa, sprinkle of onion, and garlic powder	½ Milk
⅓ cup carrot sticks, ⅓ cup celery sticks, 3 bell pepper rings, slice of kohlrabi or jicama	¾ Vegetable

Dinner

Baked potato stuffed with ½ cup kidney beans and onions, topped with 1 ounce grated part-skim mozzarella	2 Grain/Starch 1 Grain/Starch-½ Protein 1 Protein
¾ cup Bibb lettuce, 1 black olive, purple onion rings, 1 tablespoon low-calorie Italian dressing	1 Vegetable ½ Fat
½ cup steamed Swiss chard with squeeze of lemon	1 Vegetable
1 cup nearly frozen melon balls or chilled watermelon	1 Fruit
1 cup skim milk	1 Milk

1,350—DAY 2

Breakfast

Strawberry milk: blend 1¼ cups strawberries, ¾ cup skim milk; pour over ¾ cup Nutri-Grain flakes and ¼ cup All-Bran or Bran Buds (or serve cereal and milk topped with strawberries)

1 Fruit
¾ Milk
1½ Grain/Starch

Snack

½ cup steamed asparagus spears, 1½ teaspoons mayonnaise

1 Vegetable
1½ Fat

Lime-flavored sparkling water, 7 dried apricots

1 Fruit

Lunch

⅛ 15-inch vegetable pizza (4-ounce slice), whole wheat crust

2 Grain/Starch, 1 Protein, 1 Fat

1 cup shredded romaine lettuce, ½ cup spinach leaves, ½ cup alfalfa sprouts, ⅓ cup chopped tomato, 4 cucumber slices, 3 black olives, 2 tablespoons sunflower seeds, 1 tablespoon low-calorie Italian dressing

2½ Vegetable

½ Fat
1 Protein-1 Fat
½ Fat

1 orange

1 Fruit

Dinner

2½ ounces broiled trout with lime juice, sliced green onion, dill, garlic, paprika

2½ Protein

1 cup Boston lettuce, ¼ cup chopped celery, 2 tablespoons chopped bell pepper, 1 tablespoon low-calorie French dressing

1½ Vegetable
½ Fat

⅔ cup baked butternut squash, pinch of cardamom

1 Grain/Starch

¾ cup steamed broccoli with sliced water chestnut

1½ Vegetable

3 ounces no-alcohol red wine or unsweetened apple-raspberry juice

½ Fruit

Snack

¾ cup fresh pineapple pieces

1 Fruit

Snack

3 cups air-popped popcorn with ½ tablespoon grated Parmesan

1 Grain/Starch

1,350—DAY 3

Breakfast

2 whole grain pancakes (for crepes), ⅓ cup unsweetened crushed pineapple, 2 tablespoons part-skim ricotta

1 Grain/Starch-1 Fat
1 Fruit, ½ Protein

¾ cup skim milk with ¼ to ½ teaspoon instant decaffeinated coffee powder

¾ Milk

Lunch

Tuna salad sandwich: 2 slices multigrain bread, ¼ cup tuna or salmon mixed with 1 tablespoon chopped bell pepper or celery, 1 tablespoon low-fat yogurt, 4 chopped walnut halves	2 Grain/Starch 1 Protein 1 Fat
4 cherry tomatoes, ¼ pickle, purple onion rings	½ Vegetable
1 cup skim milk, 1 banana	1 Milk, 2 Fruit

Snack

½ small papaya (1 cup) topped with 3 tablespoons low-fat yogurt, 1 tablespoon peanut butter, 2 tablespoons Bran Buds or Grape Nuts, 1 teaspoon molasses	1 Fruit, ¼ Milk 1 Protein-1 Fat

Dinner

1 cup whole wheat ribbon noodles, ⅓ cup tomato sauce heated with 3 tablespoons part-skim ricotta, pinch of cayenne	2 Grain/Starch 1 Vegetable 1 Protein
¾ cup steamed spinach or 1¼ cups spinach salad	1½ Vegetable
½ cup steamed summer squash with pearl onions, ½ teaspoon margarine	1 Vegetable ½ Fat
1 slice whole wheat garlic French bread, ½ teaspoon margarine	1 Grain/Starch ½ Fat
Mint tea, 1 fresh fig or 6 fresh cherries	½ Fruit

1,350—DAY 4

Breakfast

1 scrambled egg, ⅓ cup diced tomato, 1 sliced green onion	1 Protein ½ Vegetable
1½ ounces **Breakfast Sausage** or 1 ounce 95% fat-free ham	1½ Protein
1 whole grain English muffin, ½ teaspoon margarine, 1 tablespoon apple butter	2 Grain/Starch, ½ Fat ½ Fruit
Decaffeinated tea with spoonful skim milk	

Lunch

3 to 4 ounces sliced grilled tofu with reduced-sodium soy sauce or Worcestershire sauce, garlic and onion powder, mustard or cayenne; or 1 ounce Monterey Jack	1 Protein
Half rye bun or 1 slice pumpernickel rye	1 Grain/Starch
1 cup cold steamed cauliflower, carrots or squash, and broccoli or green beans, ½ cup steamed zucchini and snow peas, 6 sliced mushrooms, 1½ teaspoons safflower oil, sprinkle of wine vinegar, marjoram	3½ Vegetable 1½ Fat
1 cup skim milk, 1 teaspoon molasses	1 Milk

Snack

Whole wheat bran muffin	1 Grain/Starch-1 Fat
1 cup skim milk, 1 plum	1 Milk, ½ Fruit

Dinner

²/₃ cup **Hearty Black Beans**, 2 corn tortillas	1½ Grain/Starch-½ Protein 2 Grain/Starch
¾ cup shredded romaine lettuce, ½ sliced tomato, 1 tablespoon sliced avocado	1 Vegetable ½ Fat
Manzanilla (chamomile) tea, 2 tangerines	1 Fruit

1,350—DAY 5

Breakfast

¾ cup 100% bran or 1 cup oat bran flakes, 1½ chopped prunes	1½ Grain/Starch 1 Fruit
1 cup skim milk	1 Milk

Lunch

3 ounces snapper filet baked with 1 tablespoon
  low-fat yogurt, ½ tablespoon whole grain
  cracker crumbs, 1 teaspoon grated Parmesan,
  paprika; or 2 ounces lean, breaded fish sticks
	3 Protein

Baked Fries, 1 tablespoon ketchup	2 Grain/Starch
Cabbage slaw: ¾ cup grated purple cabbage, 3 tablespoons low-fat yogurt	1 Vegetable ¼ Milk
½ cup steamed carrots and parsley	1 Vegetable
½ cup steamed okra with diced tomato, or steamed green beans	1 Vegetable
Spiced herb tea	

Snack

2 tablespoons toasted unsalted sunflower seeds	1 Protein-1 Fat
½ cup grapefruit juice	1 Fruit

Dinner

½ cup whole grain macaroni topped with 1 ounce grated Cheddar, paprika	1 Grain/Starch 1 Protein
½ cup lima beans with sprinkle of imitation bacon bits	1 Grain/Starch

1¾ cups shredded romaine and ¼ cup head
  lettuce, 1 radish, 1 tablespoon low-calorie
  French dressing
	2 Vegetable
	½ Fat

1 cup cantaloupe wedges, ¼ sliced kiwi	1 Fruit
Club soda with squeeze of lemon	

Snack

1 gingersnap	½ Grain/Starch
1 cup skim milk, 1 teaspoon molasses	1 Milk

Breakfast

1 slice multigrain bread, grilled with 2 tablespoons low-fat cottage cheese, 1 tablespoon grated Swiss, ⅛ teaspoon sesame seeds	1 Grain/Starch 1 Protein
½ sliced banana in ½ cup orange juice	2 Fruit

Lunch

1 cup split pea soup (¾ cup split peas, ¼ cup skim milk or broth), pinch of cayenne	1½ Grain/Starch-½ Protein ¼ Milk
1 slice pumpernickel rye or whole wheat bread	1 Grain/Starch
1 cup spinach leaves, ¾ cup alfalfa sprouts, 2 tomato wedges, sliced radish and mushroom, yogurt dressing: ¼ cup low-fat yogurt spiced with 1 teaspoon lemon juice, garlic, dill, paprika, pinch of dry mustard	2 Vegetable ¼ Milk
¾ cup skim milk	¾ Milk

Snack

Banana-berry smoothie: blend ¾ cup skim milk or low-fat yogurt, ½ banana, 4 blackberries or strawberries, 6 almonds, ½ teaspoon honey	¾ Milk 1½ Fruit 1 Fat

Dinner

2½ ounces lean pork or lamb chop, 3 tablespoons unsweetened applesauce	2½ Protein ½ Fruit
½ cup brown rice, ½ tablespoon pine nuts	1½ Grain/Starch, ½ Fat
¾ cup chopped endive, ¼ cup shredded romaine lettuce, 4 tomato wedges, 1 tablespoon fine-chopped pumpkin seeds, 1 tablespoon low-calorie Russian dressing	1½ Vegetable 1 Fat ½ Fat
¾ cup baked acorn squash with cinnamon	1 Grain/Starch
½ cup steamed Brussels sprouts with lemon mustard	1 Vegetable
Iced herb tea	

Snack

1 cup sparkling water flavored with 2 tablespoons low-calorie cranberry juice, lemon peel

Breakfast

Banana French toast: dip 2 slices firm whole grain bread in ½ cup skim milk, 1 beaten egg, and ½ mashed banana; sauté in 1 teaspoon margarine; top with ½ cup **Festive Fruit Sauce:** ¾ cup raspberries or strawberries, ¼ cup blueberries	2 Grain/Starch ½ Milk, 1 Protein 1 Fruit, 1 Fat 1 Fruit
Decaffeinated coffee with ¼ teaspoon vanilla	

Snack

³/₄ cup carrot and celery sticks, sliced cucumber	1 Vegetable
1 Swedish rye cracker (¹/₂ ounce)	¹/₂ Grain/Starch
6 ounces low-sodium tomato juice, dash Tabasco	1¹/₂ Vegetable

Dinner

2¹/₂ ounces baked "fried" chicken, light and dark meat (skinned), dipped in buttermilk and 3 tablespoons crushed Nutri-Grain flakes, 1¹/₂ teaspoons brewer's yeast, thyme, garlic, pinch cayenne	2¹/₂ Protein
³/₄ cup mashed potatoes with 1 tablespoon skim milk, ¹/₂ teaspoon margarine	1¹/₂ Grain/Starch ¹/₂ Fat
²/₃ cup steamed broccoli with lemon juice	1¹/₂ Vegetable
¹/₃ cup corn and ¹/₄ cup green peas with pimiento	1 Grain/Starch
1 whole wheat and bran dinner roll	1 Grain/Starch

Snack

Fresh sliced peach with ¹/₄ cup low-fat yogurt, 1 teaspoon molasses or honey, pinch of cinnamon or ginger	1 Fruit ¹/₄ Milk

Snack

1¹/₂ graham crackers with 1 tablespoon almond butter, 2 tablespoons raisins	¹/₂ Grain/Starch, 1 Fat 1 Fruit
1 cup skim milk	1 Milk

1,650—DAY 1

Breakfast

2 Shredded Wheat biscuits, ¹/₂ sliced banana	2 Grain/Starch, 1 Fruit
³/₄ cup skim milk	³/₄ Milk

Snack

Oat bran muffin	1 Grain/Starch-1 Fat
Sangrita: ¹/₂ cup low-sodium tomato juice, ¹/₂ cup orange juice, squeeze of lime	1 Vegetable 1 Fruit

Lunch

Chalupas: 2 corn tortillas crisped in oven and topped with ²/₃ cup mashed pinto beans, 1¹/₂ ounces grated part-skim mozzarella, hot salsa or jalapeño slice	2 Grain/Starch 1¹/₂ Grain/Starch-¹/₂ Protein 1¹/₂ Protein
¹/₂ large sliced tomato, 2 to 3 romaine lettuce leaves, 2 tablespoons sliced avocado, 2 tablespoons chopped pumpkin seeds	¹/₂ Vegetable 1 Fat 1 Protein-1 Fat
Ginger soda: club soda with 1 tablespoon lemon juice, ¹/₈ to ¹/₄ teaspoon ginger, artificial sweetener; or 1 light beer	(2 Fat)

Dinner

3 ounces roast chicken leg and thigh (skinned), basted with 1 tablespoon tomato juice, white wine, or lemon juice, tarragon, garlic; 3 tablespoons **Low-Fat Gravy**	3 Protein
½ cup mashed potatoes, 1 tablespoon **Low-Fat Gravy**	1 Grain/Starch
½ cup steamed cauliflower and carrot strips with sliced mushroom	1 Vegetable
½ cup steamed asparagus with 1 tablespoon lemon juice	1 Vegetable
1 whole wheat dinner roll, 1 teaspoon margarine	1 Grain/Starch, 1 Fat
4 ounces dry white wine (if no beer today)	(2 Fat)

Snack (if no wine or beer today)

Baked apple with 1 tablespoon low-fat yogurt, ½ teaspoon molasses or maple syrup, allspice, cinnamon	1 Fruit
¾ cup skim milk	¾ Milk

1,650—DAY 2

Breakfast

2 whole wheat nut and bran muffins, 2 tablespoons part-skim ricotta	2 Grain/Starch-2 Fat ½ Protein
Fresh fruit salad: ½ cup orange sections, ½ sliced banana, 8 fresh cherries or strawberries, 2 tablespoons pineapple juice, kiwi slice	3 Fruit
1 cup skim milk	1 Milk

Snack

1 whole wheat pretzel	1 Grain/Starch
1 tablespoon dry-roasted unsalted mixed nuts	1 Fat
6 ounces low-sodium tomato juice	1½ Vegetable

Lunch

Steamed veggies: ⅔ cup broccoli, ½ cup cauliflower, ¼ cup zucchini and mushrooms, red or yellow bell pepper strips, basil, garlic	3 Vegetable
1 cup whole wheat or spinach pasta topped with 1 ounce grated provolone, ¼ cup chopped parsley	2 Grain/Starch 1 Protein
Hibiscus tea	

Dinner

1 cup black-eyed peas	2 Grain/Starch-1 Protein
2-inch cube whole grain corn bread	1 Grain/Starch-1 Fat
⅓ cup steamed kale and ¼ cup chopped turnip greens, or ½ cup steamed spinach; ¼ cup diced turnips, 2 pearl onions	1½ Vegetable
Hot decaffeinated tea with lemon peel	

Snack

Eggnog Custard   1 Protein, 1 Fruit,
                                         2 Milk

1,650—DAY 3

Breakfast

1½ slices multigrain toast, ½ teaspoon   1½ Grain/Starch, ½ Fat
   margarine
1⅓ cups cantaloupe wedges with 2 tablespoons   1½ Fruit
   low-fat cottage cheese, 6 grapes or blueberries   ½ Protein
Decaffeinated coffee with cinnamon stick

Lunch

Tuna salad: 3½ tablespoons (1½ ounces) tuna, 2   1 Protein
   tablespoons green peas, 1 tablespoon low-fat
   yogurt, ½ tablespoon reduced-calorie   ½ Fat
   mayonnaise, ½ tablespoon sunflower seeds   ½ Fat
¾ cup shredded romaine lettuce, ⅓ cup grated   2 Vegetable
   carrots, ⅓ sliced cucumber, 6 sliced
   mushrooms, 3 tablespoons chopped parsley, 2
   tablespoons grated yellow squash, 1 tablespoon
   chopped sunflower seeds, sprinkle vinegar   1 Fat
3 rye crispbread crackers (1½ ounces)   1½ Grain/Starch
1 cup skim milk, 1½ teaspoons molasses   1 Milk

Snack

½ cup low-fat yogurt, ¼ cup unsweetened   ½ Milk, ½ Fruit
   applesauce, 4 tablespoons granola   1 Grain/Starch-1 Fat
5 mini rice cakes or 1 brown rice cake   ½ Grain/Starch

Dinner

Spinach crepes: 2 whole grain pancakes or thin   1 Grain/Starch-1 Fat
   tortillas, ½ cup steamed or thawed frozen   1 Vegetable
   spinach, 1 ounce grated part-skim mozzarella, 1 Protein
   4 tablespoons part-skim ricotta or low-fat   1 Protein
   cottage cheese, sprinkle of garlic, pinch of
   nutmeg and cayenne
¾ cup baked acorn squash with grated orange   1 Grain/Starch
   peel
½ cup sliced beets or tomato marinated with 1   1 Vegetable
   tablespoon low-calorie Italian dressing   ½ Fat
Lime-flavored sparkling water

Snack

⅓ cup Bran Buds or All-Bran, 1 sliced banana   1 Grain/Starch, 2 Fruit
¾ cup skim milk   ¾ Milk

1,650—DAY 4

Breakfast

1 poached or fried egg, no added fat	1 Protein
1 whole wheat bagel, 2 teaspoons low-sugar or 100% fruit jam	2 Grain/Starch 1/2 Fruit
1 cup skim milk, 1/2 grapefruit	1 Milk, 1 Fruit

Lunch

2 cups garden vegetable soup: 1/2 cup red beans, 1/3 cup barley or brown rice, 1/3 cup carrots and celery, 1/4 cup cabbage, 2 sliced mushrooms	1 Grain/Starch-1/2 Protein 1 Grain/Starch 1 1/2 Vegetable
2 to 4 whole wheat crackers (1 ounce)	1 Grain/Starch
Fresh pear half with 1/3 cup low-fat cottage cheese, 3 chopped Brazil nuts (1 tablespoon)	1 Fruit, 1 Protein 1 Fat

Snack

1/3 cup oysters (3 ounces), or 1/2 ounce Gruyere, or 8 shrimp (2 ounces)	1 Protein
2 Swedish rye crackers (1 ounce)	1 Grain/Starch
Perrier with lime	

Dinner

Lentil-sesame burgers: form into patties and pan-bake 1/2 cup cooked lentils, 5 tablespoons chopped parsley, 4 sliced mushrooms, 2 tablespoons sesame seeds, 1 tablespoon chopped onion; serve with Dijon mustard	1 Grain/Starch-1/2 Protein 1/2 Vegetable 1 Protein-1 Fat
1/3 cup grated carrots, 2 Bibb lettuce leaves, 2 celery sticks, 1/2 radish	1/2 Vegetable
1/2 cup steamed cauliflower, 1 tablespoon grated Cheddar	1 Vegetable 1/2 Protein
Steamed artichoke, 1 tablespoon reduced-calorie mayonnaise or 1 1/2 tablespoons sour cream	2 Vegetable 1 Fat
Apple tea: 3/4 cup decaffeinated tea, 1/4 cup apple juice	1/2 Fruit

Snack

3 **Chris's Kringles** cookies	1 Grain/Starch, 1/2 Fruit 1/2 Fat
1 cup skim milk	1 Milk

1,650—DAY 5

Breakfast

2 slices whole wheat toast with 1 tablespoon raisins, 1 teaspoon margarine	2 Grain/Starch 1/2 Fruit, 1 Fat
Orange Snow	1 Fruit, 1 1/2 Milk

Lunch

Muffin pizzas: split multigrain English muffin, 2 tablespoons tomato paste, 1 ounce grated part-skim mozzarella, 2 teaspoons grated Parmesan, 2 sliced mushrooms, bell pepper rings, sprinkle of oregano and garlic	2 Grain/Starch 1 Vegetable 1½ Protein
¾ cup spinach leaves, ½ cup shredded romaine lettuce, ⅓ sliced cucumber, 1 teaspoon grated Parmesan, sprinkle of herb vinegar	1½ Vegetable
1 cup skim milk, 1 cup nearly frozen grapes	1 Milk, 1 Fruit

Snack

3 cups air-popped popcorn, ½ tablespoon reduced-calorie margarine melted with 1½ teaspoons brewer's yeast, ⅛ teaspoon chili powder or taco seasoning, sprinkle of garlic, pinch of salt	1 Grain/Starch 1 Fat
Club soda with orange slice	

Dinner

Far East stir fry: 3 ounces pork tenderloin or beef round strips, 1½ cups sliced cabbage, broccoli, and bean sprouts, ½ cup snow peas and celery, 5 sliced mushrooms, 1 sliced water chestnut, 1 tablespoon cashews, 1 tablespoon sesame oil	3 Protein 4½ Vegetable 1 Fat 3 Fat
1 cup steamed brown rice	3 Grain/Starch
Mandarin orange tea, 1 fortune cookie	½ Grain/Starch

Snack

¾ cup fresh pineapple spears ⅓ cup blackberries	1½ Fruit

1,650—DAY 6

Breakfast

1 whole wheat waffle, topped with ½ ripe persimmon and ½ mashed banana, or 1 banana, or 1 tablespoon real maple syrup, or 3 to 4 tablespoons artificially sweetened maple syrup, and 2 tablespoons low-fat yogurt spiked with vanilla	1 Grain/Starch-1 Fat 2 Fruit
1 cup skim milk	1 Milk

Lunch

Tofu hamburger: 2 to 2½ ounces lean ground round, 2 ounces crumbled tofu, ¼ cup chopped onion, ¼ cup chopped celery, 2 sliced mushrooms, Worcestershire sauce, dash of soy sauce, multigrain bun	3 Protein ½ Vegetable 2 Grain/Starch

½ cup alfalfa sprouts, ⅓ sliced tomato, ¼ cup Boston lettuce leaves, pickle slice, purple onion rings, mustard	1 Vegetable
½ cup steamed summer squash with onions	1 Vegetable
½ cup steamed collard greens, sprinkle of vinegar	1 Vegetable
Cranapple fizz: ⅓ cup unsweetened cranberry-apple juice, ½ cup sparkling water	½ Fruit

Snack

4 apricots or 1 peach, 6 almonds	1 Fruit, 1 Fat

Dinner

1¼ cups whole grain spaghetti	2½ Grain/Starch
½ cup tomato sauce with ⅔ cup broccoli, 2 tablespoons diced eggplant, 4 sliced mushrooms, 1 tablespoon grated Parmesan, 1 tablespoon chopped pumpkin seeds	3½ Vegetable ½ Protein 1 Fat
1 cup spinach leaves, ½ cup shredded romaine lettuce, 2 teaspoons olive oil, sprinkle of red wine vinegar	1½ Vegetable 2 Fat
½ cup steamed carrots with basil	1 Vegetable
2 whole wheat bread sticks	1 Grain/Starch
Ice water with mint, squeeze of lemon	

Snack

Carob cocoa: 1 cup skim milk, 1½ tablespoons carob powder, ½ to 1 teaspoon molasses or honey, ⅛ teaspoon cinnamon	1 Milk ½ Fruit
4 animal crackers	½ Grain/Starch

1,650—DAY 7

Breakfast

1 cup hot oat bran cereal or ¾ cup old-fashioned oatmeal, 4 chopped dried apricots, 1 tablespoon raisins	1½ Grain/Starch 1 Fruit
¾ cup skim milk	¾ Milk

Snack

1 hard-cooked egg	1 Protein
1 small undercooked potato, sliced and crisped in oven, sprinkled with chili seasoning, hot salsa, or seasoned salt	1 Grain/Starch
½ cup grapefruit juice with ¼ cup unsweetened pineapple juice	2 Fruit

Lunch

Bean-spread pita: ½ cup mashed garbanzo or other cooked beans, 1 tablespoon sesame tahini, 2 teaspoons lemon juice, 1 teaspoon brewer's yeast, sprinkle of garlic, pinch of cayenne, spread in 2 whole wheat pita halves (1½ ounces bread); top with ⅓ cup shredded carrots, ¼ cup chopped tomato, ¼ cup alfalfa sprouts, 2 tablespoons chopped cucumber, 1 tablespoon chopped purple onion

1 Grain/Starch-½ Protein
1 Fat

1½ Grain/Starch
1 Vegetable

Cherry-flavored sparkling water

Snack

1 ounce Swiss cheese, 1 whole grain cracker (¼ ounce)

1 Protein

1 orange

1 Fruit

Dinner

Shrimp or chicken creole: sauté 3 tablespoons chopped celery, 3 tablespoons chopped onion, and 1½ tablespoons chopped bell pepper in 2 teaspoons olive oil; combine with 2½ ounces cooked shrimp, ¾ cup canned tomato, ½ cup sliced okra, ⅓ cup frozen corn, bay leaf, garlic clove

½ Vegetable
2 Fat
1 Protein
2 Vegetable
1 Grain/Starch

1 cup brown rice

3 Grain/Starch

Lemon-mint tea

Snack

Raspberry whip: blend ¾ cup strawberries, ½ cup unsweetened raspberries, ¾ cup skim milk or buttermilk, artificial sweetener to taste

1 Fruit
¾ Milk

2,000—DAY 1

Breakfast

Bean burritos: 2 corn or whole wheat tortillas, ½ cup mashed black or pinto beans

2 Grain/Starch
1 Grain/Starch-½ Protein

1 cup fresh papaya or cantaloupe cubes

1 Fruit

Snack

Pineapple Oat Bran Muffin

1 Grain/Starch-1 Fat

½ cup skim milk or low-fat yogurt, ⅛ teaspoon vanilla

½ Milk

Lunch

Chef salad: 2 ounces light and dark turkey, 1
ounce part-skim mozzarella or 4 tablespoons
low-fat cottage cheese, 1 cup shredded
romaine or leaf lettuce, ³/₄ cup spinach leaves,
¹/₃ cup diced tomato, ¹/₃ cup shredded cabbage,
¹/₄ cup grated carrots, bell pepper strips, ¹/₄
cup croutons (from oven-dried whole grain
bread), 2 tablespoons sunflower seeds, 1¹/₂
tablespoons vinegar and olive oil dressing
4 to 6 whole wheat crackers (1¹/₂ ounces)
Iced herb tea, 1 apple

2 Protein
1 Protein
3 Vegetable

1 Protein-1 Fat
1¹/₂ Fat
1¹/₂ Grain/Starch
1 Fruit

Dinner

Pea and Potato Curry: 1¹/₂ cups vegetables,
¹/₂ cup low-fat yogurt
2 ounces flatbread or whole grain pita
Ice water with squeeze of lemon

1 Grain/Starch, 2 Vegetable,
2 Fat, ¹/₂ Milk
2 Grain/Starch

Snack

Tapioca: heat and stir 1 cup skim milk and 3
tablespoons tapioca granules until thick; add
¹/₂ sliced banana, 1 teaspoon molasses or
honey, ¹/₈ teaspoon vanilla
3 graham crackers

1 Milk
1¹/₂ Grain/Starch
1 Fruit

1 Grain/Starch

2,000—DAY 2

Breakfast

Cinnamon toast: 2 slices whole wheat bread, 1¹/₂
teaspoons margarine, 1¹/₂ teaspoons molasses
or honey, ¹/₄ teaspoon cinnamon
Wake-up smoothie: blend ¹/₂ cup skim milk, 1
small egg, ¹/₂ cup orange juice, ¹/₂ banana, ¹/₄
teaspoon vanilla

2 Grain/Starch
1¹/₂ Fat

¹/₂ Milk, 1 Protein
2 Fruit

Lunch

Stuffed tomato-pepper: scoop out 1 medium
tomato and 1 small bell pepper; fill with ¹/₂
cup hot cooked lentils, top with 1¹/₂ ounces
grated Swiss or provolone, dash of hot salsa,
and heat through
¹/₂ cup bulghur pilaf, couscous, or brown rice
with 2 tablespoons chopped parsley, diced
tomato (or combine bulghur and lentils)
2 Swedish rye crackers (1 ounce)
1 cup skim milk, 2 small pears

1¹/₂ Vegetable
1 Grain/Starch-¹/₂ Protein
1¹/₂ Protein

1 Grain/Starch

1 Grain/Starch
1 Milk, 2 Fruit

Dinner

1½ cups chicken-noodle soup: 1½ ounces chicken breast (skinned), ½ cup whole grain alphabet noodles, ¼ cup chopped celery	1½ Protein 1 Grain/Starch
2 whole wheat biscuits	2 Grain/Starch-2 Fat
½ cup shredded romaine lettuce, ½ cup spinach leaves, sliced radish, green onion, 2 tablespoons low-fat yogurt with dill and garlic	1 Vegetable
½ cup steamed green beans with oregano	1 Vegetable
½ cup steamed carrots with ginger or summer squash with onions (or add veggies to soup)	1 Vegetable
½ cup fresh or frozen blueberries	½ Fruit

Snack

2 brown rice cakes spread with 4 tablespoons part-skim ricotta, 2 chopped fresh or dried figs, 2 tablespoons fine-chopped filberts, 1 teaspoon toasted coconut, sprinkle of cinnamon	1 Grain/Starch, 1 Protein 1 Fruit 1 Protein-1 Fat
¾ cup skim milk	¾ Milk

2,000—DAY 3

Breakfast

1 cup Nutri-Grain flakes, 2 tablespoons raisins	2 Grain/Starch, 1 Fruit
¾ cup skim milk plus 1 tablespoon nonfat dry milk	¾ Milk

Snack

2 egg rolls	2 Grain/Starch, 2 Vegetable, 1 Fat
1 cup orange-grapefruit juice	2 Fruit

Lunch

Peanut butter sandwich: 2 slices whole wheat bread, 2 tablespoons peanut butter, 4 sliced strawberries, 1 small sliced kiwi	2 Grain/Starch 2 Protein-2 Fat 1 Fruit
1 cup skim milk	1 Milk

Snack

3 Swedish rye crackers (1½ ounces) with 1 ounce melted part-skim mozzarella	2 Grain/Starch 1 Protein
⅔ cup raw carrot and celery sticks, kohlrabi slice	1 Vegetable

Snack

1¾ cups chilled watermelon	1½ Fruit

Dinner

Cookout kabobs: 2 ounces sea scallops, 2 ounces lean beef round, 6 cherry tomatoes, ¼ cup pearl onions, ½ sliced bell pepper, ¼ cup unsweetened pineapple chunks, 4 mushrooms; baste with Worcestershire or soy sauce, unsweetened pineapple juice, vinegar, garlic	3 Protein 2 Vegetable 1 Fruit
2 ears corn on the cob, 2 teaspoons margarine	2 Grain/Starch, 2 Fat
⅔ cup brown rice with 2 pineapple chunks, scallions	2 Grain/Starch
¾ cup ice milk or 3 small whole grain cookies	1 Grain/Starch-1½ Fat
Sugar-free ginger ale or lemon-flavored sparkling water	

2,000—DAY 4

Breakfast

Scrambled tofu: 3 ounces tofu, 1 egg, 1 tablespoon skim milk	2 Protein
1½ whole grain English muffins, 1½ teaspoons margarine	3 Grain/Starch, 1½ Fat
1 cup honeydew wedges, 6 fresh cherries or ⅓ cup strawberries	1½ Fruit
Decaffeinated coffee with 1 teaspoon molasses	

Snack

Maple-nut yogurt: ¾ cup low-fat yogurt, 4 black walnut halves, 1 to 1½ teaspoons molasses or real maple syrup, pinch of ground cloves	¾ Milk 1 Fat
3 graham crackers	1 Grain/Starch

Lunch

Baked potato topped with 2 tablespoons low-fat yogurt, 1 teaspoon grated Parmesan, lemon juice, garlic, chives, paprika	2 Grain/Starch
⅔ cup adzuki or navy bean chili with onion	1½ Grain/Starch-½ Protein
¾ cup **Cheryl's Sunflower Slaw**	2 Vegetable, 1 Fat
¾ cup skim milk	¾ Milk

Dinner

1½ cups baked spaghetti squash, 4 tablespoons low-fat cottage cheese, 4 tablespoons part-skim ricotta, 2 tablespoons tomato paste, 2 tablespoons sunflower seeds, ¼ teaspoon oregano, sprinkle of cinnamon	3 Vegetable, 1 Protein 1 Protein 1 Vegetable 1 Protein-1 Fat
¾ cup steamed spinach with nutmeg or 1¼ cups spinach salad with mushrooms	1½ Vegetable
2 slices whole wheat garlic French bread	2 Grain/Starch
Grape soda: ½ cup grape juice, ½ cup sparkling water	1 Fruit

Snack

¾ cup Nutri-Grain cereal or 1 whole wheat bran muffin with ½ cup strawberries, 2 chopped dates	1½ Grain/Starch 1½ Fruit
½ cup skim milk	½ Milk

2,000—DAY 5

Breakfast

1 whole rye bagel, 2 tablespoons part-skim ricotta or 2 teaspoons Neufchatel	2 Grain/Starch ½ Protein
Fresh fruit salad: ½ cup strawberries, ⅓ cup orange or apple slices, ⅓ cup unsweetened canned or fresh pineapple chunks, ⅓ cup grapes, ¼ cup low-fat yogurt, squeeze of lemon	2 Fruit ¼ Milk
Hot herbal tea	

Snack

12 **Tortilla Chips**, hot salsa	2 Grain/Starch
6 tablespoons **Spicy Guacamole**	2 Fat

Lunch

¾ cup lima beans with ¾ ounce extra-lean ham pieces	1½ Grain/Starch 1 Protein
2 whole grain corn muffins	2 Grain/Starch-2 Fat
1½ cups shredded romaine lettuce, ½ cup spinach leaves, ¼ cup shredded carrots, ¼ cup diced tomato, 2 tablespoons chopped parsley, 1½ tablespoons Thousand Island dressing	2½ Vegetable 1½ Fat
1 cup skim milk	1 Milk

Snack

Coffee yogurt: ½ cup low-fat yogurt, 1½ teaspoons real maple syrup or honey, ¼ teaspoon instant decaffeinated coffee powder, ⅛ teaspoon vanilla	½ Milk ½ Fruit
2 plums	1 Fruit

Dinner

Beef or venison stew: 3 ounces lean stew meat, ⅔ cup potatoes, ½ cup green beans and carrots, ⅓ cup cabbage, ¼ cup green peas, 2 tablespoons chopped celery, 2 tablespoons chopped parsley, 1 tablespoon chopped onion, bay leaf, garlic, pinch of cayenne	3 Protein 2 Grain/Starch 2 Vegetable
2 slices sourdough rye or pumpernickel rye, 1 teaspoon margarine	2 Grain/Starch 1 Fat
½ cup skim milk, 2 small tangerines	½ Milk, 1 Fruit

2,000—DAY 6

Breakfast

²/₃ cup 100% bran or 1 cup Roman Meal cereal, ½ sliced banana, 2 chopped dates, 4 pecan halves — 1½ Grain/Starch, 2 Fruit, 1 Fat

1 cup skim milk — 1 Milk

Lunch

½ cup **Spinach Dip**, 6 cherry tomatoes, ⅓ bell pepper cut in strips, ⅓ cup carrot sticks, ⅓ cup steamed asparagus, ¼ cup cucumber slices, 1 mushroom — ½ Protein, 1 Vegetable, 2½ Vegetable

4 medium sardines (2 ounces), mustard, horseradish — 2 Protein

3 Swedish rye crackers (1½ ounces) — 1½ Grain/Starch

1 orange — 1 Fruit

Lemonade: 1 cup sparkling water, 1 tablespoon lemon juice, ½ tablespoon honey, sprig of mint — ½ Fruit

Snack

Happy hour: 6 ounces club soda, 2 dashes angostura bitters, lemon wedge

3 tablespoons (1 ounce) dry-roasted unsalted mixed nuts — 1½ Protein-1½ Fat

Dinner

Spanish rice: sauté 2½ tablespoons chopped onion and 1 tablespoon chopped bell pepper in 1 teaspoon soybean oil; add 3 tablespoons canned tomatoes, 1 teaspoon hot salsa, ⅔ cup cooked brown rice — ½ Vegetable, 1 Fat, 2 Grain/Starch

1 cup pinto beans with ¼ cup chopped cilantro or parsley — 2 Grain/Starch-1 Protein

2 corn or whole wheat tortillas — 2 Grain/Starch

½ cup chayote, Mexican summer squash, or yellow squash — 1 Vegetable

4 tablespoons mashed avocado on 1 slice tomato, 1 lettuce leaf — 2 Fat

½ fresh mango or 1 cup melon, chilled — 1 Fruit

¾ cup skim milk or iced peppermint tea — ¾ Milk

Snack

1 slice whole grain melba toast (from oven-dried pumpernickel rye or whole wheat bread) or 1 whole grain pancake, 1 tablespoon part-skim ricotta — 1 Grain/Starch

Passion punch: ⅓ cup passion fruit juice or apple-raspberry juice, ½ cup sparkling water — 1 Fruit

2,000—DAY 7

Breakfast

Potato pancakes: form two patties from ½ cup stiff, mashed cooked potato, ½ beaten egg, 2 tablespoons chopped onion; sauté in 1 teaspoon margarine or oil; top with ¼ cup unsweetened applesauce, 1 tablespoon cranberries or ½ tablespoon cranberry sauce, ¼ cup low-fat yogurt

1 Grain/Starch
½ Protein

1 Fat
½ Fruit

¼ Milk

¾ cup skim milk, 6 ounces prune or pineapple juice

¾ Milk
2 Fruit

Snack

2 whole wheat blueberry-bran muffins

2 Grain/Starch-2 Fat

1 fresh peach, ¼ cup cottage cheese

1 Fruit, 1 Protein

Lunch

Pasta and pine nuts salad: ¾ cup whole wheat spirals, 3 tablespoons canned garbanzo beans, ⅔ cup chopped tomato, ⅓ cup steamed asparagus or artichoke hearts, ⅓ cup steamed broccoli, ¼ cup snow peas, ¼ cup red bell pepper strips, 1 sliced mushroom, 2 sliced green onions, 1 sliced black olive, ½ tablespoon grated Parmesan, ½ tablespoon pine nuts, 1 tablespoon olive oil, 2 teaspoons red wine vinegar

1½ Grain/Starch
½ Grain/Starch
3 Vegetable

½ Fat
3 Fat

Orange-flavored sparkling water

Dinner

3 ounces liver with onions

3 Protein

1 baked sweet potato (½ cup) or 1½ cups baked acorn squash, pinch of allspice

1 Grain/Starch

¾ cup steamed broccoli, squeeze of orange and lemon juice, ½ tablespoon chopped cashews

1½ Vegetable
½ Fat

½ cup steamed cauliflower with paprika

1 Vegetable

2 whole wheat dinner rolls, 1 teaspoon margarine

2 Grain/Starch, 1 Fat

Decaffeinated tea

Snack

3 cups air-popped popcorn with cinnamon

1 Grain/Starch

⅓ cup mixed dried fruit (figs, apples, dates, pears, apricots, or raisins)

2 Fruit

1 cup skim milk, 1 teaspoon molasses

1 Milk

2,300—DAY 1

Breakfast

Egg and potato tacos: 2 corn or whole wheat tortillas, 1 scrambled egg, ½ cup diced, steamed potatoes, hot salsa	2 Grain/Starch 1 Protein 1 Grain/Starch
½ grapefruit, strawberry garnish	1 Fruit
6 ounces prune or grape juice	2 Fruit
Decaffeinated coffee	

Lunch

Roast beef sandwich: 2 slices pumpernickel rye, 2 ounces lean beef, ½ ounce part-skim mozzarella, 1 teaspoon mayonnaise, leaf lettuce, purple onion ring, mustard	2 Grain/Starch 2½ Protein 1 Fat
⅔ cup steamed green beans	1½ Vegetable
⅔ cup corn with pimientos	1½ Grain/Starch
½ cup steamed kale and red cabbage with vinegar and caraway seeds	1 Vegetable
1 cup skim milk	1 Milk

Snack

Nectarine-blueberry parfait: 1 large sliced nectarine or peach, ¼ cup blueberries, ½ cup low-fat yogurt, 6 chopped almonds, 1 tablespoon Grape Nuts or toasted wheat germ, almond extract, cinnamon, ginger	1 Fruit ½ Milk 1 Fat
2 whole wheat raisin-bran muffins	2 Grain/Starch-2 Fat
1 cup skim milk	1 Milk

Dinner

1 cup whole grain noodles, ½ cup tomato sauce with ¼ cup chopped parsley, 1½ ounces part-skim mozzarella, ½ tablespoon grated Parmesan	2 Grain/Starch, 1 Vegetable 1½ Protein
2 slices whole wheat French bread	2 Grain/Starch
½ cup steamed eggplant with garlic and ½ tablespoon grated Parmesan	1 Vegetable
½ cup steamed zucchini with basil	1 Vegetable
1½ cups shredded romaine lettuce, 1 cup spinach leaves, 2 teaspoons olive oil, sprinkle red wine vinegar	2½ Vegetable 2 Fat
6 ounces no-alcohol wine, or 3 ounces dry red wine, or 3 ounces red grape juice with sparkling water	1 Fruit

2,700—DAY 1

Breakfast

Grilled cheese: 2 slices whole grain bread, 1½ ounces Swiss cheese, caraway seeds	2 Grain/Starch 1½ Protein
1 cup hot apple cider with cinnamon stick	2 Fruit

Snack

1 slice whole wheat gingerbread	1 Grain/Starch-2 Fat
1 cup skim milk	1 Milk

Lunch

1 cup navy beans with ½ tablespoon molasses, ¼ teaspoon dry mustard; or 1½ cups navy bean soup	2 Grain/Starch-1 Protein
2 slices pumpernickel rye or Boston brown bread	2 Grain/Starch
¾ cup steamed beet greens, dash of vinegar	1½ Vegetable
½ sliced tomato	1 Vegetable
1 cup skim milk	1 Milk

Snack

Circus snacks: 1½ cups air-popped popcorn, ½ cup granola, 3 tablespoons dry-roasted peanuts, 2 tablespoons raisins	½ Grain/Starch, 2 Grain/Starch-2 Fat, 1½ Protein-1½ Fat, 1 Fruit
Banana frost: blend 1 fresh or frozen banana, ¾ cup grapefruit juice, 4 ice cubes	3½ Fruit

Dinner

3 ounces roast light and dark turkey, 4 tablespoons **Low-Fat Gravy**	3 Protein
⅔ cup whipped sweet potato in scooped-out orange cups	2 Grain/Starch
½ cup steamed green peas with mint and mushrooms	1 Grain/Starch
½ cup steamed cauliflower with lemon juice and paprika	1 Vegetable
2 whole wheat dinner rolls, 2 teaspoons margarine	2 Grain/Starch, 2 Fat
1 cup grapes	1 Fruit

Snack

Hard-cooked egg	1 Protein
Blender gazpacho: 6 ounces tomato juice, ¼ cucumber, 1 teaspoon lemon juice, garlic, dash of Tabasco, parsley sprig	2 Vegetable

✔ PRACTICE: LEAVE ONE BITE

Some kids are taught to clean their plates because of all the starving children in Africa. Others leave a bite of food for the fairies in hopes of getting a bigger prize for that tooth shoved under the pillow. But grown-ups know there are better ways to deal with world hunger than by eating too much. (They also know their lost tooth means a big bill from the dentist and no reward from the stingy fairy.) Still, established habits die slow and hard.

Just for this week, leave one bite of each food on your plate. If your only cue to stop eating is seeing the bare windmills and flowers on your bone china, this practice may be a tough one, especially at a restaurant ("I paid for it; I'm going to eat every scrap of it"). The tougher it is for you, the more subconscious significance it packs, so give it a try. After all those years of clean plates, your fairy is looking mighty hungry.

PRACTICE: REPEAT PRACTICE

"Play it again, Sam!" If the first time was only fair-to-good, give it another shot—it may be better-to-great the second time around. Replay any practice from the first five weeks that needs more work, or design a practice to suit your needs. It took a good long while to create an unproductive habit, so give yourself enough time—and enough effort—to break it.

✏️ ✅ Practice Diary Six

Although it might seem that following preplanned menus would be the easiest and most accurate way to live lean, planning your own menus—learning to make choices—or revising existing menus to fit your tastes is good on-the-eating-job experience for you. Many times you have to make instant decisions about what to eat, as when you file through a cafeteria line or when someone offers you a brownie. Keep the Good Food Guide within easy reach until you know it by heart. Once you discover how many calories are saved (and how many nutrients are earned) by making simple "good food" choices, you may have more incentive to make them more of the time.

PLAN/RECORD MEALS AND SNACKS

SUNDAY

MONDAY

TUESDAY

WEDNESDAY

THURSDAY

FRIDAY

SATURDAY

PRACTICE DIARY SIX

Practices

Practices	Day							Notes
	Su	M	Tu	W	Th	F	Sa	
Aerobic Activity—30 minutes, 4 days a week								
Plan/Record Meals and Snacks								
Personal Time Out—30 minutes, twice a day								
Leave One Bite								
Repeat Practice								

✓ = yes, I did try;　　✓✓ = yes, I did welll

Suggested Practices

- Compare your recommended daily calories with the calories you actually eat in Quantity Control Assurance.
- Create an all-purpose meal plan for yourself using the Sample Menu Design.
- Try out some of the Training Table Menu ideas this week; mix and match to suit your tastes.

GOOD FOOD GUIDE TALLY

	Gr/St	Pro	Veg	Fruit	Milk	F/HF	Extras
Sug. Daily Por.							

Sug. Daily Por. = Suggested Daily Portions (Maximum)
Gr/St = Grain/Starch　　　　　Veg = Vegetables
Pro　 = Protein　　　　　　　　F/HF = Fat/Hidden Fat

WEEK SEVEN

Stress: Fix It before You Break
   *Assess Your Stress
    Stress-Prevention Strategies
   *Stress Rx
    Practice: Take Stress in Stride
    Where Have All the Hours Gone?
   *Take Time to *Make* Time

Speed Eating Is Not a Sport
    Practice: Slow Down and Savor

*Stalking Simple Sugars
    Shakedown on Sugar
    Choosing a Sweetener
    Practice: Slack Off on Sweets

*Practice Diary Seven

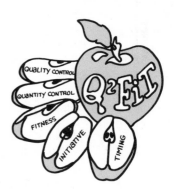

Stress: Fix It before You Break

Larry is an executive in a multinational computer company. His reward for taking his career too seriously is an angry hole in the lining of his stomach. When it flares up, it's hard for him to eat a balanced meal, let alone a balanced diet. When it subsides, he still craves alcohol, the only thing that helps him relax after a killer day.

Nancy holds a high-level position with a communications corporation. "I really love my job," she maintains. But her year-end bonus for such dedication consists of high blood pressure, elevated blood cholesterol, allergic hives, chronic exhaustion, and compulsive eating. During the Living Lean project she came to an unhappy conclusion: "I have to admit it; my job is destroying me."

A good portion of Larry's and Nancy's stress is not demanded by the boss or spelled out in a job description. Rather it's self-imposed—"I ought to do this" or "I am expected to do that." When Nancy began leaving work early (5:30 P.M.) so she could join a fitness class, no one said a word. "They sit there working like slaves and don't even notice when I leave. I feel terribly guilty." Not to mention it's tough when you discover you aren't indispensable.

If you try to do it all, and do it all well, you can look forward to plenty of physical and emotional sacrifice. Three-fourths of visits to family doctors and internists (who often deal with odd and assorted health problems) are related to unrelieved stress, with diagnoses ranging from allergy, acne, alcoholism, and backache to migraine, insomnia, colitis, and depression. If you are secretly grateful when you have to ring up the boss to call in sick, take a hint; reduce the stress or your body will do it for you—the only way it knows how.

Some people get so hooked on a high-pressure life they no longer recognize the stress they endure. "I'm used to it—I can take it." Persistent side effects like hypertension, ulcers, high blood cholesterol, and chronic infections insist other-wise. Other physical stress effects just compound the health problems—sodium and water retention, impaired digestion, enhanced blood clotting, increased blood sugar, muscle protein breakdown (loss of lean), and food cravings—especially for the Spoilers sugar, salt, caffeine, and alcohol. Even if you manage to ignore the cravings and eat only high-quality foods, stress still works against you by depleting important nutrients like vitamin A, vitamin C, pantothenic acid, potassium, cal-cium, magnesium, zinc, iron, copper, and more.

So what does stress have to do with Living Lean? Look back over these physi-cal effects and real-life stories, and see how often eating or drinking are inter-twined with stress. When their tails are pinched, laboratory rats immediately re-spond to the stress by eating. If you feel like *your* tail is being pinched on a regular basis, you can constantly grapple with a runaway appetite or you can do something about the stress.

The problem is, we have few socially acceptable channels for the little angers, frustrations, or energy slumps that are part of the average workday. An employee who rests his head on his desk with eyes closed may be viewed as lazy or goofing off. But the lunch hour is sacred (except for a terminal workaholic), to be filled up as he or she pleases—usually with eating and drinking. Nor would a conscientious parent indulge in a hot bath while there are hungry mouths to feed. But half a box of Girl Scout cookies can be wolfed down while simultaneously taking care of the dinner chores.

The following exercise might help pinpoint what's eating you—and also what you're eating in response.

✐ ASSESS YOUR STRESS

- Using the chart on page 146, write down all the things that are causing stress, tension, anger, or unhappiness for you right now. They can be major frustrations, like a financial crisis or a constant feeling of loneliness; or minor, picky things that really annoy you, like a car that breaks down or a family member who throws bath towels on the floor. Keep in mind that anything extreme or unusual (moving to a new apartment, severe weather, chronic noise, grief, even monotony) can be con-sidered stressful.
- Now rank them in order of importance; little irritations can be high on the list. Decide whether each will be important next week, next month, or next year (some problems tend to disappear on their own).
- Were any of the same situations responsible for your eating (or drinking) too much, especially when you weren't particularly hungry, as noted on your Eating Diary?
- Indicate who (including yourself) or what is causing the stress. Regardless of the source, describe *what* you can do about it and *how* you can do it.
- Now list several of your current goals—for your career, your relationships, your self-fulfillment. Are any of the stresses interfering with your Living Lean goals?

Avoiding stress is the easiest route. For instance, if you invariably gobble up the cookies you keep for unexpected guests, stop buying them; if a co-worker thrives on argument or makes cutting remarks, respond with a noncommittal "um-hmm" or "Some people feel that way," and then leave.

Try to communicate to solve the problem, or change the situation if you can't avoid it. When your mother criticizes your eating habits or your appearance, ex-plain how it hurts your feelings and makes you resentful, thus less likely to change;

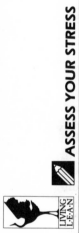

ASSESS YOUR STRESS

| Stress or problem | Priority ranking | Will it still be important in | | | Eating related? | Who or what is responsible? | What can I do? How? | Current goals |
		1 wk.?	1 mo.?	1 yr.?				

if you and your spouse don't communicate on an issue, draft a referee or an arbitrator and set some ground rules: "I'll try to do this better if you'll try to do that better."

If you can't escape or improve the situation, you'll have to cope with it. Instead of going bananas, go away occasionally—even if you have to hire a babysitter for a day; if a relative is intent on self-destruction with alcohol and rebuffs treatment, visit Al-Anon so you don't go under, too.

If you don't do this whole exercise, merely list your current stresses and add to your list during the next few days.

WHAT'S YOUR PLEASURE?

Diagnose the malady to select the remedy:

- If your life is boringly predictable, do something frivolous or unexpected— give a gift for no reason, take an unplanned excursion.
- If you're up to your eyebrows in brain work, do something physical— clip the hedges, go jogging or dancing.
- If you're feeling unorganized, clean out a closet or storeroom and put it back together so you can find everything.
- If you've been existing on TV dinners, cook up a special dish or eat out at a really great restaurant.
- If your life has been chaotic, do something orderly—work on needle-point or a jigsaw puzzle.
- If your job is making you sick and miserable, seek another one and rediscover your lost health and happiness.
- If your life seems unimaginative, read a book of adventure or fantasy.
- If you are lost in a tangle of details and can't seem to focus on what's important, go someplace with an unlimited view—the beach, the mountains, the desert—and expand your horizons.
- If everyday problems get blown out of proportion, volunteer to help those less fortunate.

STRESS-PREVENTION STRATEGIES

People who blame fate or others for their troubles often feel stuck when they find themselves in a stressful situation. Jane is a good example: "My boss has never offered me a raise." "If I don't pick up my teenagers' clothes, they stay on the floor." "I love to walk, but my husband won't go with me at night, and I have to get the kids ready for school in the morning." "I only have a half hour for lunch, so I end up with fast food or a cola and candy bar from the vending machine." "I'm doomed to be overfat—it's in my genes." Hold on. Who's in charge here? Unless Jane initiates some changes, it's obvious changes will not be made. And she does have some options.

Several of the following stress-preventing philosophies helped Jane as she attempted to regain control of her life. If any appeal to you, list them on your Practice Diary this week.

- Eat nutritious foods and snacks on a regular schedule when you're under stress.
- Aerobic activity and plenty of sleep are good antidotes for a hectic workday.

- Avoid the Spoilers; sugar, salt, caffeine, and alcohol can add to stress rather than relieve it. (One study found a brisk walk relieved stress and tension for several hours, while a candy bar aggravated it, and rather quickly.)
- There's nothing as therapeutic as getting it off your chest. Find a good listener.
- Patience is a virtue—slow down.
- Become thick-skinned about criticism—opinions are not facts.
- Much of the pressure on you (to be a good mother, a good provider, a good student) is self-imposed.
- Those who seek perfection are guaranteed failure. Give yourself credit for what you have accomplished rather than worrying about what you haven't accomplished.
- Avoid making too many changes (a new job, a new marriage) all at once.
- Overexpressing anger can be as physically destructive as bottling it up. Don't waste your stress hormones unnecessarily.
- Anticipating trouble (dental anxiety, for example) is often worse than the trouble itself.
- When a situation reaches the boiling point, it often initiates badly needed changes. Things have a way of working out for the best.
- If you're stuck in a "can't cope" situation, try prayer. You might not get exactly what you want, but you will get just what you need.

STEP OUTSIDE

Fresh air, sunshine, tranquility. You get more than an aerobic workout when you play outdoors, and these side effects may be just as important for your health, according to recent research. For instance, some people get depressed, chronically sleepy, and ravenously hungry—especially for sweets and chocolate—during the winter. Doctors say they suffer from SAD (seasonal affective disorder), and the prescribed therapy is increased activity and exposure to bright indoor light for several hours each day. It's probably no accident that popular vacation spots are sunny and cheery, not cloudy, foggy, or gloomy!

If you simply feel like bobbing on a swim float or swinging in a hammock today instead of jogging around the park, you will still reap some of the rejuvenating side effects of outdoor activity.

How many outdoor hours do you log a week? _____

Can you plan a 30-minute sunshine and fresh-air break every day?

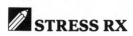 **STRESS RX**

Once your littlest angel spills nail polish on the new carpet, it's too late for stress prevention. Instead of popping a tranquilizer (in this case, a Twinkie), substitute one of these quick stress solutions to ease the tension before it gets totally out of hand. (If time is scarce, the starred items are particularly fast and effective.) Add one or two Stress Rx ideas to your Practice Diary, or devise some of your own.

- a tall glass of ice water with lemon; a cup of herb tea
- a nutritious snack

- a short walk; a long walk or run
- a nap or extra hours of sleep
- vigorous sweeping or cleaning, mowing the yard, or washing the car
- yoga, meditation, a relaxation tape
- slow, deep breathing
- lying flat on the floor for 5 minutes (a bed or couch works, too, but the floor is especially effective)
- a massage or tension-relieving stretches, particularly for neck and shoulders or feet
- a cold foot soak (in summer), a warm foot soak (in winter)
- a long shower or bath; a soak in a whirlpool
- a TV show; radio or stereo music
- complete silence
- a book, magazine, or movie; an engaging hobby
- a romp with children or a pet; a get-together with friends
- complete solitude
- just sitting outdoors in a serene place

Your Ideas

ARE YOU BREATHING?

Well, of course you're breathing, but are you *really* breathing? Or is a mere thimbleful of air flowing in and out right now?

You can easily fix that, plus give your brain an invigorating shot of oxygen at the same time. Put your hand on your abdomen; it should expand when you breathe in and contract when you breathe out. Now count to five as you slowly breathe in, and five again as you breathe out. Next time you're caught in traffic, angry at the kids, nervous about public speaking, or just tired of sitting, try deep, slow breathing. It's almost as good as taking a walk.

✅ PRACTICE: TAKE STRESS IN STRIDE

Being stressed out all the time doesn't feel very good, and it can really hamper your Living Lean progress. On your Practice Diary, list one or two of the top stresses from Assess Your Stress, plus your proposed remedies from Stress-Prevention Strategies and Stress Rx. Rehearse any special techniques ahead of time, and memorize how it feels to be completely relaxed and carefree. Even a little stress saved is a lot of tranquility earned.

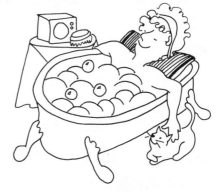

Put Stress to Rest

WHERE HAVE ALL THE HOURS GONE?

Some people chase fame, others chase fortune, but the new grand prize in our hurry-up world is time—enough time to do the many things we want to do. No doubt you're glad not to have to grow all your own food, beat your laundry on a rock, or make the children's clothing by hand. But would you find time to stitch and piece a quilt these days, or just sit in the porch swing and contemplate life? Even with smaller families and more conveniences, it's hard to take time out for such luxury these days. Where do all the hours go?

Mostly they go to work. During the past 15 years you have lost one-third of your leisure time; that's 520 fewer hours a year, gobbled up by career and chores. Automation and technology promised to save our leisure time from such a fate, but all they have really saved is calories. Then, too, we may be suffering from assembly-line syndrome. Whenever we save a few minutes, we feel obliged to do more and do it faster. Rapid transportation and communication allow us to see more than seven countries in a week; or to cram a score of appointments into an average workday. But crowding and fragmenting our time never seems to make us feel that we have more time. And according to Living Lean students, "I don't have time" is the primary roadblock to living a lean life.

TAKE TIME TO *MAKE* TIME

If a hectic schedule is crowding out things you really want to do—or must do—take time to sit down with a pencil right now and *make* time. Very briefly, outline when things happen in a typical day, in between your scheduled meal and snack times. Don't forget time for getting to work, getting home, cooking and chores, aerobic activity, family fun or communication time, as well as your time all to yourself. Analyze, revise, consolidate, and eliminate. If you're stumped, show your itinerary to someone and ask for suggestions.

TYPICAL SCHEDULE

Time	Activity
_____	Wake up
_____	Breakfast
_____	Snack
_____	Lunch
_____	Snack
_____	Dinner
_____	Go to bed

Take Time to Make Time

✎ "I WISH I HAD ENOUGH TIME TO . . . "

If you can honestly say "Yes, I do try" to these questions, indicate with a check (✓).

☐ If things are not satisfactory as they are, do you set a few reasonable goals and make necessary changes to work toward them?

☐ Since it's impossible to do everything—and do it well—do you choose one or two goals as priorities? (A crowded life is not necessarily a rich life.)

☐ If you can't start at the beginning of a big project and finish it, do you start somewhere, then go back and fill in the gaps later?

☐ Do you avoid the deception of rushing (to work, to get finished) so you'll have more time to relax?

☐ Do you delegate work, at home as well, if you are shouldering more than your share? Do you ask for help on a project when you need it?

☐ Can you politely say "no" and feel positive rather than guilty about it?

☐ Do you eliminate excess stuff from your life—possessions, unnecessary chores, meaningless routines? Can you find what you need when you need it?

☐ Can you create a few minutes of personal peace even in the midst of hustle and bustle—daydreaming on the bus, enjoying a hobby, reading in the tub, a leisurely walk during the lunch hour?

☐ Do you have at least one meal each day that is relaxed, seated, business-free, and rejuvenating? Preferably two? Ideally three?

☐ Are you comfortable with unplanned time? (Doing nothing is not the same thing as wasting time.)

☐ Do you allow for creative or relaxation time during the day, with a sunshine and fresh-air break if possible? Do you take short breaks often?

☐ Do you seek out people—family, friends, strangers—to enrich your daily life? Do you spend enough time with them?

☐ Do you have a date to do something special with your friend, spouse, or child every week? Do you look forward to social engagements rather than wondering how you're going to fit them in?

☐ Do you consider vacations, little and big, as necessities rather than luxuries? Do you plan some fun during the week as well as on the weekend?

☐ When you work hard to acquire things to make your life enjoyable (camping gear, antiques to refinish), do you set aside enough time to enjoy them?

Speed Eating Is Not a Sport

"You eat too fast, Bruce."

"What difference does it make? The same food still goes down the hatch whether I eat it fast or slow." Only that's not necessarily so.

A University of Alabama study found that high-fiber foods took longer to eat—15 extra minutes per day, to be exact—and the result was a daily decrease of 1,500 calories. It takes 20 to 30 minutes for your stomach to send a message to your brain, saying, "Okay, Mac, we're finally getting some food down here. Slow down on fuel loading." If you can choke down an enormous number of calories in only 13 minutes flat, then you completely miss out on your body's natural "overfill prevention" mechanism. On the other hand, if you extend your average eating time, you are more likely to get full before your plate is empty, thus consuming fewer calories.

You might want to try a couple of these tricks to slow your aerobic-style eating. They don't take much conscious effort.

- If tension causes you to eat too fast, take a few minutes before the meal is served to relax or take a few deep breaths.
- Serve dinner before it's ready. Begin with soup, vegetable appetizers, or a salad. While you're chatting and digesting the first course, waiting for the second course to get done, the satiety signals have time to shut down excessive hunger.
- Serve high-volume foods and beverages before or with your meal: peppermint herb tea, sparkling water with a squeeze of lemon, homemade soup. Studies have found lower-calorie vegetable, noodle, bean, or broth soups to be just as satisfying—and filling—as higher-calorie cream or cheese soups.
- Eat high-fiber foods that require lots of biting and energetic chewing: heavy breads, hearty crackers, popcorn, raw vegetable salads.
- For fun, use chopsticks for your main meal or a fork or spoon for finger foods like sandwiches, chicken, and cookies.

Here are a few techniques that require a little more conscious attention.

- Play a secret game—be the last one to finish eating without relying on second helpings. (Be sure no one else at the table is playing the same game!)
- If you eat alone, look at your watch and try to stretch your snacks to 5 or 10 minutes and your meals to 20 minutes or more.
- Pretend this meal is the last of your food rations for a while. Stretch it out—take small bites and chew thoroughly, noticing the crunch, the aroma, the flavor, and the temperature of what's in your mouth.
- While you're chewing your food, try putting your fork or spoon down. Concentrate on the current bite, not the next one.
- Try eating in front of a mirror. Do you look relaxed? Try not to bend over your plate, shoveling your food down. Instead, "fork-lift" it to your mouth (it takes longer that way).

Let's face it: when we have exceeded the point of "pleasantly hungry," we eat like starved animals—fast and without thinking. Hark back to the Hunger Busters (Chapter 2) if your every meal looks like an Olympic speed-eating contest.

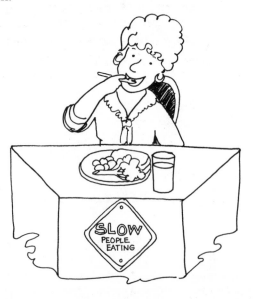

Slow Down and Savor

✔️ PRACTICE: SLOW DOWN AND SAVOR

It's bad enough when you can't remember what you had to eat for lunch today, much less what you ate yesterday. But it's still worse when you eat so fast you don't even get a good look at your food. ("No, officer, I don't remember what color the popsicle was.") What's the big rush?

If you'd like, add at least one, or perhaps two, of the slow-down ideas to your Practice Diary. Try to determine how long it takes your hunger meter to shut off. Write yourself a few "slow" memos. This is the week of the snail; savor your meals and enjoy your prime dine time.

📝 Stalking Simple Sugars

When Mom gave you your first taste of a cookie, somehow you knew it was love at first bite. Ever since then, the endearing days in your life have come packaged with enduring sweets—birthday cakes, Valentine's Day candy, Christmas cookies—and it's just not the same without them. Sweets and love walk hand in hand, and if you're too shy to give a hug or a kiss, a sweet treat will deliver your message just the same.

Intentionally or unintentionally, your sweet tooth has been sharpened over the years. We eat 500 percent more sugar today than we did in the 1800s—126 pounds (25 five-pound bags) of sugar per year. That's a half cup or 450 calories each day and a whopping 18 percent of our total calorie intake.

"But I hardly ever eat desserts." "We don't even have a sugar bowl." Still, you could be taking in several hundred calories of white lightning every day without knowing it: 60 percent of the sugar you eat comes hidden in sweet (and not-so-sweet) processed foods. Did you know 25 percent of the calories in pork and beans and cream-style corn are sugar? For All-Bran, it's 29 percent; Dannon low-fat fruit yogurt and Carnation Instant Breakfast, 37 percent; Quaker Instant Maple Oatmeal, 35 percent; Nature Valley Granola Clusters, 50 percent; and ketchup and relish, 63 percent. Like spy dust, it's hard to track down the source because the label doesn't have to tell you how much there is.

Even an all-American meal may offer otherwise nutritious fare laced with sucrose or corn syrup additives. In this menu, test your sugar savvy by circling the foods that are not likely to contain added sweeteners.

Granola and milk	Peanut butter
Cranberry juice cocktail	Graham crackers
Raisin toast and jelly	Pork sausage with barbecue sauce
Coffee with nondairy creamer	French fries with ketchup
Fruit yogurt	Baked beans, canned peas
Ham sandwich	Lettuce with French dressing
Tomato soup, sweet pickle	Lemonade
Cole slaw	
Canned peaches	

If you selected milk, coffee, french fries, and lettuce, you're correct. The central question is, do you really want to eat your daily sugar concealed in ketchup, salad dressing, and canned peas? All those hidden teaspoons could be traded in for an oatmeal cookie—maybe a couple of 'em.

On the other hand, 40 percent of your usual sugar is visible to the naked eye. Soft drinks, syrup, jelly and jam, gelatin desserts, slushy drinks, popsicles, and table sugar are major suppliers, with cakes, cookies, pies, and pastries following close behind. Now let's check your sugar savvy in the "sweet treats" category.

Foods in the following list are obviously sweet, but what isn't always clear is which have more sugar and which have less. Put a check mark (✓) by the "winner" in each pair. (The answers are given in number of teaspoons so you can fill in sugar amounts for each item and use this chart as a reference. Note: 1 teaspoon sugar = 15 calories.)

Food	Serving	Sugar (teaspoons)
1. Cola soft drink	12 ounces	_____
Orange soda	12 ounces	_____
2. Cranberry juice cocktail	8 ounces	_____
Gatorade	8 ounces	_____
3. Ginger ale or tonic water	12 ounces	_____
Root beer	12 ounces	_____
4. Apple butter	1 tablespoon	_____
Jam or jelly	1 tablespoon	_____
5. Chewing gum, hard candy, jelly beans	1 piece	_____
Saltwater taffy	1 piece	_____
6. Fudge or chocolate candy bar	1 ounce	_____
Granola bar	1 ounce	_____
7. Sweetened applesauce	½ cup	_____
Canned peaches, light syrup	½ cup	_____
8. Angel food or sponge cake	2½ ounces	_____
Yellow cake with icing	3½ ounces	_____
9. Glazed doughnut	1½ ounces	_____
Chocolate brownie with nuts	1 ounce	_____
10. Sugar cookie	2	_____
Oatmeal cookie or gingersnap	2	_____
11. Fig bar	2	_____
Graham cracker	2	_____
12. Cherry or apple pie	⅟7 pie	_____
Pecan pie	⅟7 pie	_____
13. Lemon or chocolate chiffon pie	⅟7 pie	_____
Pumpkin pie	⅟7 pie	_____
14. Chocolate fudge topping	2 tablespoons	_____
Whipped topping, pressurized	2 tablespoons	_____
15. Ice cream	1 cup	_____
Ice cream sundae	1 cup	_____
16. Sherbet	1 cup	_____
Fruit yogurt	1 cup	_____
17. Chocolate milk	8 ounces	_____
Thick milkshake	11 ounces	_____
18. Jell-O or chocolate pudding	½ cup	_____
Tapioca	½ cup	_____

Answers

1.	10	4.	1½	7.	4½	10.	3	13.	9½	16.	13½
	12		3		2½		1½		3½		6
2.	6½	5.	½	8.	6½	11.	2½	14.	4	17.	3
	3½		1		9		1		½		9½
3.	8	6.	3½	9.	2	12.	4½	15.	11½	18.	4
	10½		1½		2½		12		19		3

When you're eating anyone else's version of cake, pie, or cookie—be it Auntie Alice's or Sara Lee's—your best and perhaps only clue to the recipe comes from your sweet taste buds. Once you untrain them by cutting down on desserts or experimenting with low-sugar alternatives, they'll grow happier with less. Then spread the enlightenment; volunteer to bring the dessert to a club meeting or church supper, and be sure to let your eating audience know you baked it with their health in mind, using less sugar as well as high-fiber, low-fat ingredients. (Maybe they'll catch on and return the gesture: "Cook unto others as you'd like them to cook unto you.")

SOME SWEET THINGS

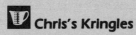

Chris's Kringles

A college student who brought a tin of these cookies to class one night went home empty-handed. Nowadays people are tuned in to treats that are both good-tasting and good for them as well.

½ cup oatmeal
½ cup whole wheat flour
¾ cup raisins
1 teaspoon cinnamon
1 teaspoon allspice
¼ teaspoon nutmeg
½ teaspoon ground cloves

½ teaspoon baking soda
1 teaspoon vanilla
1 tablespoon honey
2 tablespoons light vegetable oil
⅔ cup unsweetened applesauce
1 unbeaten egg

Combine dry ingredients. Add other ingredients and mix well. Drop by teaspoons on a lightly oiled cookie sheet, or use a nonstick spray. Bake at 350 degrees for 15 minutes or until light brown. If you like, substitute 2 packages of artificial sweetener (equivalent to 4 teaspoons sugar) in place of the honey. Makes 24 small cookies.
3 cookies = 1 Grain/Starch, ½ Fruit, ½ Fat

Festive Fruit Sauce

A fruit sauce is multipurpose: your pancakes, crepes, ice milk, or plain yogurt will love the addition.
Briefly puree 1 cup unsweetened fruit—blueberries, strawberries, apricots, canned pineapple, or mixed fruit—in the blender. Makes about ½ cup.
¼ cup for mixed fruit, ½ cup for berries only = 1 Fruit

SHAKEDOWN ON SUGAR

"Sugar isn't so bad. After all, an ounce of fudge has fewer calories than a large apple." But the resemblance ends there. Unlike the apple, sugar is fiber-free, and a second glance through the list of Sweet Treats reveals most of the foods it tags along with won't win acclaim for fiber either. Thus, you can eat more before you start to feel full.

Fiber-bare calories from a breakfast of toasted white bread, jam, fruit juice, a sweet roll, or sugar-coated cereal are likely to hit your bloodstream like a mild jolt of electricity. Blood sugar may soar too high, too fast. This elbows your pancreas to release the hormone insulin. Insulin's job is to take sugar out of blood and put it into cells, where it can be processed for energy or stored as fat. If you are watching the morning soaps instead of pounding the sidewalks while reveling in jelly dough-nuts, the sugar calories will most likely head for a final resting place in your fat depot.

A couple of hours later, the energy boom may give way to an energy bust. For some people, the combined insulin peak plus blood sugar slump triggers hunger for more super-sweet stuff—just in time for the morning coffee-and-pastry break—and the roller coaster cycle starts all over again. (Those who complain of feeling weak or tired quite soon after indulging in sweets may actually be experiencing "brain drain." Sugar attracts large volumes of water to the intestine, lowering the blood volume and shorting the brain's blood supply.)

Most people don't suffer from severe blood-sugar swings, thank goodness. But sugar is still a Spoiler, either provoking hunger for more sweets you don't need ("I can't believe I ate that whole bowl of pudding") or canceling your appetite for foods you do need—"spoiling" your dinner, as Dad used to say. While it's crowding whole-some foods out of your repertoire, sugar provides zilch in the vitamin-mineral de-partment. It also hastens the loss of calcium, zinc, chromium, and possibly other nutrients from your body. Of 20 patients with diagnosed symptoms of thiamin defi-ciency (insomnia and upset stomach, fatigue and mental confusion, irritability and uncoordination), 12 habitually consumed lots of sweet drinks, candy, and processed snack foods. Therapy was straightforward: replace refined foods with nutrient-dense choices to put thiamin back on the table.

Some nutritionists believe sugar isn't the real villain; rather, it's the sleazy company it keeps. Look through the list of Sweet Treats one more time. Many are also fat-filled, and dietary grease is another nutrient-poor, high-calorie food dis-placer. (If it weren't for sugar, though, the fat attack would lose its appeal. Can you imagine gorging on bitter baking chocolate or a sour lemon cream pie?) Still more bad company: though you'd never guess it, salt often rides shotgun alongside sugar. A half cup of chocolate pudding or an orange danish roll has more sodium than 15 saltine crackers.

No fiber, no vitamins, no minerals. Hidden fat, secret salt, erratic hormones, and excessive hunger. Specs like these may explain why sugar can foul up your body's natural metabolic setpoint, producing a gain in fat that is stubbornly resis-tant to change. Rats consistently opt for dessert (sugar) when it is offered alongside standard rat chow—and then grow fatter on the same number of calories as a result. (For humans, one *extra* soft drink a day is worth 17 extra fat-pounds in a year—a pound every three weeks!) Is sugar more fattening than high-fiber carbohy-drates? Very likely. Sugar isn't so bad in moderation, but it isn't that great either. When in doubt, leave it out.

DECREASE YOUR DIABETIC LIABILITY

Too much sugar on the table doesn't necessarily cause too much sugar in the blood, a characteristic of diabetes. But recent government studies indicate up to one-fifth of the general population—more than 30 million people—may not metabolize sugar properly. If the same people are also overfat, they are at increased risk of becoming diabetic as they grow older, especially when diabetes runs in the family.

Diabetics are more prone to developing heart disease than are nondiabetics, and the fructose component in table sugar, as well as fructose corn syrup in processed foods, may exacerbate the condition. For one thing, fructose is linked to copper deficiency, which can cause cardiac muscle damage. In susceptible people, fructose elevates uric and lactic acids, blood triglycerides, and cholesterol, while it lowers HDL levels. And these effects are all compounded by eating saturated fat.

Sugar also displaces chromium, part of the important glucose tolerance factor that declines in diabetics and older folks. Interestingly, there is ample chromium in sugar cane but not in refined table sugar, and plenty in whole wheat bread but little in refined white flour bread.

Statistics indicate 80 percent of diabetics are overfat. By cutting refined calories from fat, alcohol, and sugar and by increasing aerobic activity and dietary fiber, many diabetics have burned excess body fat, lowered blood pressure, decreased blood lipids, reduced insulin levels, and improved glucose metabolism. And for a nondiabetic, a similar plan could prevent an innocent spare tire from progressing to a diabetic liability.

CHOOSING A SWEETENER

The quick fix for our terminal sweet tooth (or so advertisers tell us) is to substitute fake sugar for the real thing. Are they right? Perhaps not. Living Lean students say they never really lose the yen for sweets as long as they have sugar taste-alikes to fall back on. Once they get hooked on reduced-calorie desserts, it's harder to turn down the real thing. Another negative of the powders and potions is the "Oh, poor me" psychological impact of being "on a diet" all the time. Then again, are you on a diet if you chug "diet" cola, then top the meal off with chocolate cheesecake?

The main reason people opt for sugar subs over simple sugar is to cut calories and obstensibly burn fat. A study of 80,000 American women found that those who used artificial sweeteners tended to gain weight over a year's time while those who didn't use them stayed the same. So much for the latter notion. Plus, when animals are given saccharin, their insulin levels increase, they end up hungrier, and they eat more. If your body thinks a sweetener is sugar, in some ways it might as well be sugar. Cutting calories this way may backfire, too. Overfat volunteers fed aspartame ate only slightly less food but a greater percentage of their calories from fat.

So it's back to the drawing board—which is the lesser of two evils, sugar or artificial sweeteners?

Artificial sweeteners—best for your teeth; fewest calories, but not effective for fat loss; insulin response similar to sugar; possible health risk, but no agreement on whether more or less risky than ordinary sugar

Fructose, sucrose—a number of health risks; calories but no nutrients; fructose triggers less insulin response

Blackstrap molasses, sorghum syrup, rice syrup, barley malt, honey, real maple syrup—longer history and more flavor than fructose and sucrose; probably similar health risks; calories but no nutrients, except for blackstrap molasses (calcium, potassium, and iron)

Fresh fruit, dried fruit—vitamins, minerals, calories; fiber slows absorption of natural sugars

Fruit juice, concentrated fruit juice—same as fresh fruit, but loss of some nutrients, less fiber, and greater insulin response; if not diluted, concentrates have more calories

Hearing the evidence, it seems the third option might be best: moderation. It increases the safety of the "fake" sugars and decreases the calorie contribution of the real ones. One to two teaspoons of fruit jam, honey, or maple syrup on your toast, in your tea, or over your pancakes will sweeten your day without expanding your waistline.

GETTING THE BEST OF SUGAR

If sugar constantly leads you into temptation, use these strategies to counteract your sugar habit and its side effects.

1. Shop for low-sugar alternatives to your usual breakfast cereals or other products with hidden sugar. Swig diluted unsweetened fruit juice instead of soft drinks. Indulge in fresh fruit topped with plain yogurt. Buy canned fruit that brags "packed in its own juice." Serve pancakes and crepes with pureed fresh fruit sauce. And use fresh or dried fruit to sweeten baked goods and desserts.

2. If you're a kitchen whiz, try the baker's secret: substitute honey for sugar in your prize pound cake, but cut the amount in half and decrease the liquid by one-fourth; or cut the called-for sugar by one-fourth to one-half; or use a sugar substitute.

3. Sweet spices can fool your taste buds and pinch-hit for part of the sugar. Experiment with allspice, anise, cardamom, cinnamon, cloves, fennel, ginger, licorice, vanilla, and almond extract.

4. Steer clear of desserts and sweets when you are vulnerable—tired, depressed, or overhungry. Instead, practice prevention: buttress your breakfast with protein and fiber and keep your blood sugar from soaring or sinking with small, frequent meals and snacks in between. Note: high-fiber carbohydrates improve your body's handling of sugar, while any low-carbohydrate "diet" (much like our everyday American eating) makes it worse.

5. Aerobic activity is all-purpose: it helps lower blood sugar when it's too high and helps raise it when it's too low. Although training assists your body to store more glycogen (carbohydrate), it decreases your dependence on carbohydrate fuel and instead encourages fat-burning. This sugar-to-fat fuel shift is especially beneficial for diabetics, hypoglycemics, and overfat folks who poop out easily at the sweat shops, because better fat-burning (i.e., aerobic metabolism) means more endurance.

✅ PRACTICE: SLACK OFF ON SWEETS

This is a test—this is only a test. Choose three or four foods you customarily eat from this list, from the Sweet Treats chart, or from your Pantry Inventory. Enter them on your Practice Diary and make an attempt to eliminate them for a week. You might want to simultaneously dump "diet" drinks and artificial sweeteners to let your sweet taste buds temporarily rest in peace (you'd be surprised how many Living Lean students report feeling better without them). Then take up the slack with fresh, fiber-rich fruit—it will taste a lot sweeter without competition from saccharin and powdered-sugar glazes. Try out a couple of strategies from Getting the Best of Sugar because you *can* get the best of it!

- soft drinks, punch, lemonade, fruit drinks
- sugar, honey, jam, jelly, syrup, cranberry sauce
- gelatin dessert, canned fruit, fruit yogurt, fruit salad (commercial)
- cakes, cookies, pies, pastries, doughnuts
- breakfast cereals, granola bars
- banana bread, muffins, granola-style loaf breads
- ice cream, milkshakes, frozen yogurt, pudding, popsicles, whipped topping
- chocolate and chocolate drinks
- candy, gum
- dessert wine, sweet mixed drinks, liqueur
- canned foods like beans and franks, tomato soup
- relish, ketchup, French dressing

✏️✅ Practice Diary Seven

Physical and emotional stress invariably lead to poor health habits like eating too fast or too much, skipping meals, craving for sweets, or relying on coffee, cigarettes, and alcohol to rev up and calm down. In turn, poor health habits further aggravate the stress and its effects on your body. What you're eating—and what's eating you—are like sinister Siamese twins, so break the vicious cycle at every possible connection. Since a stressed-out body often prefers to burn lean muscle in preference to fat, you may discover that a healthy escape from stress can shift your Living Lean project from no-progress neutral to high-gear success.

PLAN/RECORD MEALS AND SNACKS

SUNDAY

MONDAY

TUESDAY

WEDNESDAY

THURSDAY

FRIDAY

SATURDAY

PRACTICE DIARY SEVEN

Practices

Practices	Su	M	Tu	W	Th	F	Sa	Notes
Aerobic Activity—30 minutes, 4 days a week								
Plan/Record Meals and Snacks								
Personal Time Out—30 minutes, twice a day								
Take Stress in Stride								
Slow Down and Savor								
Slack Off on Sweets								

Day

✓ = yes, I did try; ✓✓ = yes, I did welll

Suggested Practices

- Spend more time outdoors—30 minutes a day if possible, as suggested in Step Outside.
- Practice deep breathing or relaxation techniques in Are You Breathing?
- Take Time to *Make Time* in your schedule for Living Lean.

GOOD FOOD GUIDE TALLY

	Gr/St	Pro	Veg	Fruit	Milk	F/HF	Extras
Sug. Daily Por.							

Sug. Daily Por. = Suggested Daily Portions (Maximum)
Gr/St = Grain/Starch   Veg = Vegetables
Pro = Protein   F/HF = Fat/Hidden Fat

WEEK EIGHT

Whatever Works—For *You*
Your Missing Link
*Something Ventured, Something Gained

*Practice Diary Eight

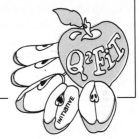

Whatever Works—For *You*

No matter what went wrong with the flight schedule, the baggage, or the reservations, Pat, an airline ticket clerk, was sure to hear about it, and then some. He usually deflected the stress with a double helping of dinner, but one day severe chest pains sent him to the emergency room, and it scared him.

He has since traded his size 42 trousers for a size 38. He attributes his health gains and fat losses to lots of fiber—fruits, veggies, and grains. "Also no caffeine, no sugar, and very little meat or fat. I eat my main meal at two o'clock in the afternoon when I get off work, and later I walk anywhere from one to two hours. It's good for me because my job is definitely high-stress. Some of my friends think I'm too thin—at size 38! But I think what they really miss is their old eating and drinking buddy. I feel absolutely great."

Darla had been overfat as long as she could remember. She desperately embraced each new "diet" as a possible salvation, but success was always fleeting, and the price she paid for it invariably too high. The side effects from one fad scheme were so severe she ended up in the hospital.

This time, however, she did it the right way, slowly and cautiously. "Changing my lifestyle habits was hard, and giving up sweets was the hardest. But I did it *for* myself, and not *to* myself. The next challenge is to stay lean, but I really respect myself for the effort I've made. And I'm not willing to sabotage that."

Both Pat and Darla made grand commitments, and they earned all-star results for their efforts. But there are less dramatic stories that need telling, too. Success comes in all shapes and sizes, and this is how it sometimes sounds:

- "After that first class, I went home and counted how many calories I actually eat. And you know what? You were right—I'm really not eating that much. At least I don't feel so guilty anymore, and I can concentrate on the other parts of the Formula that are probably more relevant for me."
- "I haven't done a lot of the things we talked about—basically I'm a lazy person. But I did buy some whole grain cereals, and I eat breakfast now, every day. I can already tell that I'm snacking less on cookies and chips between meals."
- "I didn't lose an inch over the holidays. But I didn't gain an inch either, so I'm giving myself credit for that—it's a first."
- "My problem is not enough time to organize myself to make big changes. But I am doing a few little things. For instance, instead of chips and beer at 5:30 without fail, I take a fruit break at 4:30, and that seems to hold me until dinner."
- "I know we're not supposed to weigh, but I did anyway, and this month I've only lost one scale-pound, as you call it. A few years ago, I would have considered that a failure. But this month hasn't been difficult at all—I didn't work terribly hard

at Living Lean. In fact, it's been kinda fun. So I decided if I can lose twelve pounds a year, barely trying, that's a pretty good deal."

- "Now that I'm checking my heart rate when I work out, it's obvious that I always tried to go too fast before. I'm sure that's why I never stuck with an aerobics program. I just burned out too quick."
- "Thanks for clueing me in about fat versus weight loss. My weight isn't changing much right now, but my measurements are shrinking in a hurry. If I hadn't learned about the distinction, I'd probably be discouraged right now instead of encouraged."

If you eat how you've always eaten and do what you've always done, you will feel like you've always felt and look like you've always looked. For anyone committed to Living Lean, Initiative is essential, and change is inevitable. The change sequence begins with information, progresses to inspiration, and culminates with action. You have acquired plenty of new knowledge during the past seven weeks, but are you inspired to action yet? Some folks require the entire eight weeks to get ready to begin. If you are presently dangling at the end of your inspiration, take a deep breath, close your eyes, and take a flying leap into action—it's a surprisingly easy jump. You can think big but start small, as all these men and women have done. Flip back to Chapter 1, and begin your second eight weeks using only the Practice Diaries if you wish. Trust your judgment; even before you read this book, you had a pretty good idea about what needed to be changed. In short, stop *thinking* about it, and start *going* about it!

YOUR MISSING LINK

By now, everyone who has invested a wholehearted effort in Living Lean is chalking up some success—usually in proportion to those efforts. Because of favorable changes in metabolism, even scale-pounds will start disappearing by six to eight weeks, along with the fat-pounds. The Success Formula works this way—you can count on it.

But just what if it's *not* working? What then? There is always a reason; it simply remains for you to track it down. These profiles may yield some helpful clues.

- A woman who avoided anything that even hinted of physical activity bought dozens of "diet" books, carefully counted calories, and employed special foods like "diet" drinks and desserts. She lost some weight, but remained basically overfat and out of shape.
- Another woman who suffered enormous pressures at work began a regular workout on a stationary bicycle. She never had time to eat a real breakfast or lunch; instead, a large dinner in the evening would help her unwind. Even though her total calorie intake was not excessive, her fat-burning progress was frustratingly slow.
- A man with a moderately active job started jogging to "get in better shape" when he could no longer fasten his size 34 belt. After his run, he would treat himself to cheese or chips, soda or beer, all the while wondering why he had nothing to show for his sweat except tighter jeans.

The Success Formula works but, as these examples demonstrate, only with all of its components in place. Any Missing Link has to be replaced, so how do you go about finding yours? It might be right under your nose—perhaps concealed in the chapter you decided to skip, the habit or lifestyle you felt was too difficult to change, the attitude adjustment you postponed until later. Or, you may have to do some serious prospecting to unearth it. Witness a few Living Lean students who struck gold, often where they least expected it:

- "The only thing I'm doing different is no red meat—strictly lean turkey, fish, and chicken. And it's working for me."
- "I sit with my preschoolers while they eat, but I don't join in anymore. Licking their plates clean must have been a major source of hidden calories for me."
- "My secret? I eliminated soft drinks, both regular and diet."
- "I shifted my walk to before breakfast instead of after. It seems to cut my appetite the entire day. Could that be possible?"
- "Walking every day and eating more often has made a new woman out of me. I feel wonderful. I'm on a positive roll."

Is there something you should be doing but haven't quite gotten around to yet? Is it something that will ultimately make you much happier or significantly healthier? Will it help you get lean and then make it easier for you to stay that way?

✏ SOMETHING VENTURED, SOMETHING GAINED

Jot down three positive changes you've made in your lifestyle, attitude, aerobic activity, or eating habits during your Living Lean project. Congratulations on your progress!

Next write down three changes you'd still like to make. Is one of the last three changes a potential Missing Link? What's keeping you from making it? What can you do about the holdup, and when can you do it?

Now write down one small change you *can* make, beginning today (or first thing tomorrow). Don't commit for more than one day if necessary. Then if you want, extend it for the whole week.

If all the changes aren't reward enough, now is a good time to do something really nice for yourself—you deserve it. Also write yourself a note where you can see it, or remind yourself daily: "You're doing great! Nice going. Keep up the good work."

SUCCESS: DON'T SETTLE FOR LESS

Don't forget the Success Formula. It was designed to be a helpful reminder of what makes Living Lean work, so post it where you can see it.

- Quality Control—choose foods primarily from the Good Food Guide; use caution with the Spoilers sugar, salt, caffeine, and alcohol.
- Quantity Control—select foods that are high in fiber and low in fat.
- Fitness—the most common Missing Link for Living Lean.
- Initiative—determination with a spark of enthusiasm: the "I" in Living Lean.
- Timing—eat often and you'll eat less (Quantity Control again).

Put them all together and you have Q^2FiT—the Success Formula for Living Lean. Now decide how you're going to make it work—for *you*.

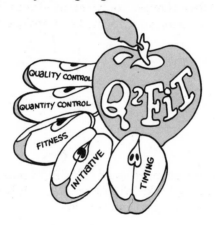

The Success Formula for Living Lean

✏️✅ Practice Diary Eight

Eight weeks! It's a long time, yet a short time in the grand scheme of things. At any rate, it's a good time to assess your progress, so flip back to the Progress Evaluation in Chapter 1 and take a second reading. Also check your measurements again (Count Down the Inches, Chapter 1). And if you'd like, fill out the Eating Diary and the Eating Diary Analysis (Chapters 1 and 2) once more. Retake the Fitness Walking Test (Chapter 3), too, if you think your fitness level has changed substantially.

You might also want to do a mirror assessment. Regardless of what the numbers say, do you look trimmer or better proportioned? Are some flabby areas becoming firmer? Are your jeans or slacks a little looser? Are your face, chin, and neck less puffy and more rosy? Do your eyes sparkle? Can you carry groceries or walk up the stairs without becoming winded? Do you have more confidence in your dealings with other people and in your ability to set goals and achieve them? Are you happier?

You can't do everything at once and do it well, so this week repeat any practice from the first seven weeks. Focus on your Missing Link if you have pinpointed it, or on particular problem areas noted earlier in this chapter in Something Ventured, Something Gained. Fitness is the key that unlocks the Success Formula for nine out of ten people, so keep moving if you don't do anything else.

Be prepared for the ups and downs in your enthusiasm—they're only natural. Read the Preface, Introduction, and Chapter 1 again if your Initiative needs a jump start. Hang on to your Treasure Map, too—your subconscious keeps working on your Living Lean project even when you aren't. If your assessment reveals you are headed in the right direction—great. Just keep up the good work. If you're making little or no progress yet, remember eight weeks of doing all the right things may not be enough time to undo many years of doing all the wrong things. Evaluate your progress after another eight weeks of Living Lean, and don't hesitate to visit a professional nutritionist if you're still stuck on square one. Good luck!

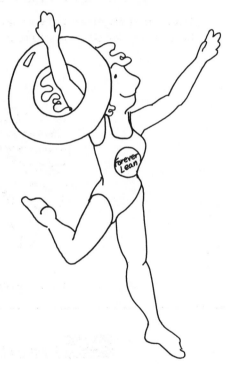

Make the Leap to Living Lean

PLAN/RECORD MEALS AND SNACKS

SUNDAY

MONDAY

TUESDAY

WEDNESDAY

THURSDAY

FRIDAY

SATURDAY

PRACTICE DIARY EIGHT

Practices	Su	M	Tu	W	Th	F	Sa	Notes
Progress Evaluation								
Count Down the Inches								
Fitness Walking Test								
Eating Diary and Analysis								
Aerobic Activity—30 minutes, 4 days a week								
Plan/Record Meals and Snacks								
Personal Time Out—30 minutes, twice a day								
Repeat Practice								

✓ = yes, I did try; ✓✓ = yes, I did well!

Suggested Practices

- Focus on particular problem areas—or your Missing Link—in Something Ventured, Something Gained.
- Keep the Q^2FiT Success Formula handy and refer to it often.
- Do a mirror assessment of your progress.
- Fitness first! Keep moving if you don't do anything else.
- Look at your Treasure Map often—it's a powerful link to your subconscious.
- Reward yourself for Living Lean—you deserve it!

GOOD FOOD GUIDE TALLY

Sug. Daily Por.	Gr/St	Pro	Veg	Fruit	Milk	F/HF	Extras

Sug. Daily Por. = Suggested Daily Portions (Maximum)
Gr/St = Grain/Starch   Veg = Vegetables
Pro = Protein   F/HF = Fat/Hidden Fat

Appendix A

BODY FAT INDICATOR SCALE

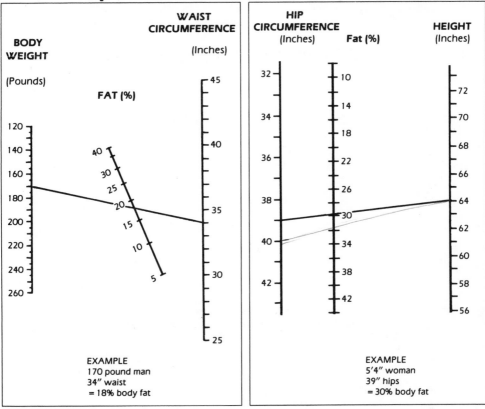

Copyright 1983 by Jack H. Wilmore, Ph.D.

To get a rough estimate (within 3 percent) of your percentage of body fat, draw a line connecting the correct values on the two outer scales. Read your fat percentage on the scale in the middle. *Note:* This estimate may not be as accurate for very lean or very overfat people.

Appendix B

THE ROCKPORT FITNESS WALKING TEST EVALUATION AND WALKING PROGRAM

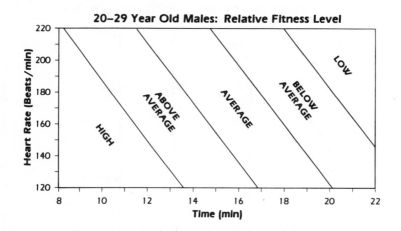

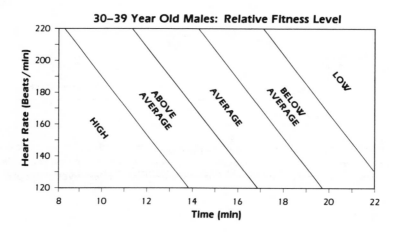

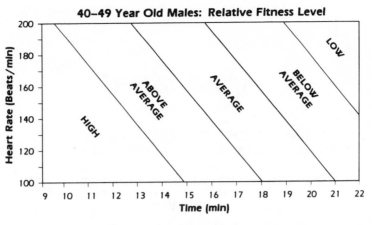

40–49 Year Old Males: Relative Fitness Level

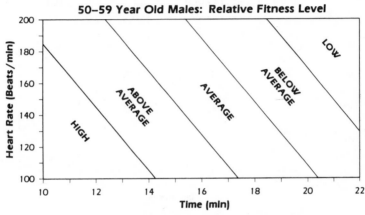

50–59 Year Old Males: Relative Fitness Level

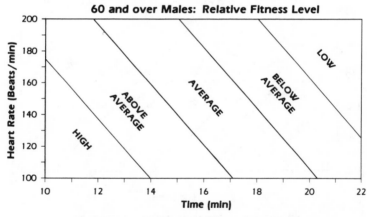

60 and over Males: Relative Fitness Level

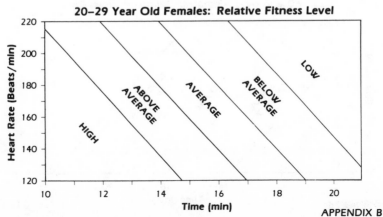

20–29 Year Old Females: Relative Fitness Level

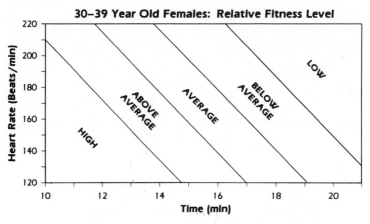

30–39 Year Old Females: Relative Fitness Level

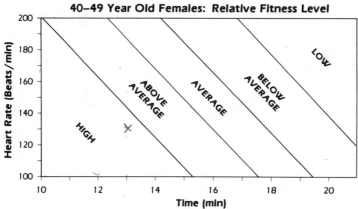

40–49 Year Old Females: Relative Fitness Level

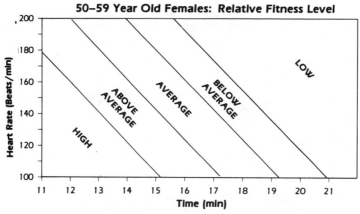

50–59 Year Old Females: Relative Fitness Level

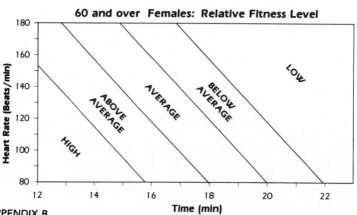

60 and over Females: Relative Fitness Level

If your relative fitness level is Low based on the Fitness Walking Test, or you are over 60, you should use the Starter Program. If your fitness level is Below Average, begin with the Starter Program. If it's too easy, skip to the Intermediate Program. If your fitness level is Average or better, begin with the Intermediate Program.

STARTER PROGRAM

Week	1	2	3	4	5	6	7	8	9	10	11	12	13	14	15	16	17	18	19	20
Mileage	1.0	1.0	1.25	1.25	1.5	1.5	1.75	1.75	2.0	2.0	2.0	2.25	2.25	2.5	2.5	2.5	2.75	2.75	3.0	3.0
Pace (mph)	3.0	3.0	3.0	3.0	3.0	3.5	3.5	3.5	3.5	3.75	3.75	3.75	3.75	3.75	4.0	4.0	4.0	4.0	4.0	4.0
Heart Rate (% of max.)	60	60	60	60	60	60–70	60–70	60–70	60–70	60–70	70	70	70	70	70	70	70–80	70–80	70–80	70–80

INTERMEDIATE PROGRAM

Week	1	2	3	4	5	6	7	8	9	10	11	12	13	14	15	16	17	18	19	20
Mileage	2.0	2.25	2.5	2.5	2.75	2.75	2.75	2.75	3.0	3.0	3.0	3.0	3.25	3.25	3.5	3.5	3.5	4.0	4.0	4.0
Pace (mph)	3.0	3.0	3.0	3.0	3.0	3.5	3.5	3.5	3.5	3.5	4.0	4.0	4.0	4.0	4.0	4.5	4.5	4.5	4.5	4.5
Heart Rate (% of max.)	70	70	70	70	70	70	70	70	70	70	70–80	70–80	70–80	70–80	70–80	70–80	70–80	70–80	70–80	70–80

Appendix C

RESOURCES

If you'd like a little more information on nutrition or fitness, here are a few reliable resources.

- For a delightful introduction to dietary fiber and its health benefits written by the physician who made fiber a household word, read *Eat Right to Stay Healthy and Enjoy Life More*, by Denis Burkitt, M.D. (New York: Arco, 1979).
- Dr. James W. Anderson and his research group offer some helpful materials on high-fiber menu planning. For information, write HCF Diabetes Foundation, P.O. Box 22124, Lexington, KY 40522.
- The colorful booklet "Exchange Lists for Meal Planning" outlines the most widely used diet-planning system. It is available for $2.00 from the American Dietetic Association, 216 W. Jackson Blvd., Chicago, IL 60606-6995.
- Tips for living well without meat (or with less meat) can be found in *Diet for a Small Planet*, 10th Anniversary Edition, by F. Lappe (New York: Ballantine Books, 1982); and in *The New Laurel's Kitchen*, by L. Robertson, C. Flinders, and B. Ruppenthal (Berkeley, CA: Ten Speed Press, 1986).
- For information on organized walking events, write the American Volkssport Association, 1001 Pat Booker Road, Universal City, TX 78148. Another resource is the WalkWays Center, 733 15th Street N.W., Washington, DC 20005. The center publishes a newsletter and provides a walker's network here and abroad.

INDEX

Accentuate the Positive, 5
Activity levels, 111–112
Activity Log, 100–101, 102
Adrenalin high, 53
Adzuki beans, how to cook, 32
Aerobic activity
    alternatives, 46–48
    benefits of, xiii–xiv, 42–43, 44, 112
    bicycling, 1, 46, 47, 55
    classes in, 45–46
    checkup before, 6
    effect of, compared to dieting, 48, 92, 112
    effect on appetite, 94–95
    effect on metabolism and muscles, 87
    Gallup survey, number of people exercising,
        viii
    heart rate monitoring during, 49–50
    jogging, 43, 46
    "killer" start-and-stop, 95
    making it fun, 53
    obstacles to, 96–97
    overdoing it, 52–53
    raising the metabolic setpoint, 90
    rationalizations against, and overcoming,
        97–98
    recommended speed, frequency, duration,
        54–55
    running, 46
    scheduling, 54, 58, 59
    strengthens bones, 106
    swimming, 46–47, 55
    symptoms of overdoing, 52
    tips for every-day activities, 98–99
    typical aerobic hour recommended, 52
    wardrobe for, 52
    See also Walking; Aerobictips
Aerobic Engineering: Move It to Lose It, 45–52
Aerobic limit, 49, 55
Al-Anon, 147
Alabama, University of, 26, 152
Alcohol, ix, 69, 104
Allergy, 6
American Dietetic Association, 174
American Medical Association, vii
American Volkssport Association, 174
Anderson, Dr. James W., 174
Anorexia, 89
Appestat, 94
Appetite control, 33–35, 94–95

Apple tea, 36
Appleseed, Johnny, 48
Are You Breathing?, 149

Bailey, Covert, Fit or Fat, 8
Baked Fries, 36
Banana French toast, 125
Banana frost, 140
Banana-berry smoothie, 125
Be an Activist!, 98–99
Bean-spread pita, 132
Beans, calcium in, 105
Beans, dried, how to cook, 32
Beans, Hearty Black, 31
Bicycling. See under Aerobic activity
Big Benefits, 42
Black beans, how to cook, 32
Black-eyed peas, how to cook, 32
Blood cholesterol, 12
Blood glucose (fasting), 12
Blood lipid profile, 6
Blood pressure, 12
Body Beautiful, 11
Body composition
    and age, 87
    changes in, 44, 87, 92
    Body Fat: Friend and Foe, 7–11
    Body Fat Indicator Scale, 169
    body fat percentage, 9–10
    effect of diet and/or aerobic activity (chart), 92
    How Much Fat is Too Much Fat?, 10
Bones, 55, 104, 106–107
Boron, 104
Brain drain, 156
Bran muffins: Pineapple Oat Bran, 31–32
Bran, wheat and oat, ways to use, 30
Breads, high-fiber kinds, 30
Breakfast Bottles and Boxes, 15
Breakfast Sausage, 77
Breastfeeding, 7
Breathing exercise, 149
Burkitt, Dr. Denis, 27, 174

Cabbage: Cheryl's Sunflower Slaw, 79
Caffeine, ix, 37–39
    amounts in various items, 38
    dangers of, 38, 104
    weaning, 39
    withdrawal symptoms, 37

Calcium, 53, 57, 73, 104–106, 145, 156
  carbonate, 105
  citrate, 105
  good sources, 104–105
Calisthenics, 45
Calories
  average adult consumption, vii
  burned while walking, 56
  equivalents, 74, 117
  in a typical restaurant meal, 76
  recommended daily consumption, 110–113
  skimping, not recommended, 7
  use of by the body, 95
Carbohydrates, 8, 26, 30
  complex and simple, 57, 66
  best fuel food, 56–57
  protein compared with, 80
Cardiovascular disease, risk of, 6
Carob cocoa, 36, 131
Cereals, high-fiber kinds, 30
Cheese, 82, 104
Chef salad, 132
Cheryl's Sunflower Slaw, 79
Chicken, baked "fried" (recipe), 126
Children, calorie-skimping not recommended
    for, 7
Chris's Kringles, 155
Chromium, 156, 157
Cinnamon toast, 133
Cocoa, carob, 36, 131
Coenzymes, 57
Coffee, amount of caffeine in, 38
Cola beverage, amount of caffeine in, 38
Comfort Equals Safety, 50–53
Complete Guide to Your Emotions, Rodale
    Press, 6
Cookies: Chris's Kringles, 155
Cookout kabobs, 135
Cooper, Dr. Kenneth, 46
Copper, 104, 105, 145, 157
Count Down the Inches, 10
Crackers, high-fiber kinds, 30
Cranapple fizz, 131
Creole, shrimp or chicken, 132
Cross-country skiing, 46
Curry, Pea and Potato, 79–80
Custard, Eggnog, 106

Dairy Delites, 106
Dessert recipes, 155
Diabetes, 6, 8, 27, 82
  decreasing your chances of, 157
  information source, 174
Dieting
  weight gain after stopping, 89
  effect of compared with aerobic activity, 48,
    92, 112
  failure of chronic, vii, ix, 1, 8, 80, 88–91, 92
  danger of low-calorie, 88
  failure of "successful," 88–91
Dried beans and peas, list of, 27
Dried beans, how to cook, 32

Eat Often (and You'll Eat Less), 35
Eating
  changing habits, 113, 151–152
  Good Food Guide, 66–83
  Living Lean options, 39
  Portion Plan, 113–119
  Ready-Made Menus, 120–140
  techniques to slow down, 152
Eating Diary, xiii, 16–17, 19
Eating Habits Checkup, 20–24
Eggnog Custard, 106
Electrolytes, 57
Enzymes, 57
Exercise. See Aerobic activity

Far-East stir fry, 130
Fat
  in Good Food Guide, 68–69, 73
  percentage of calories, 114
  saturated, 74
Fat-Skimmed Favorites, 77
Fattening foods: comparison of protein and
    carbohydrates, 80–81
Festive Fruit Sauce, 155
Fiber, 26–33, 63
  effect on digestive tract, 27
  The Fiber Connection: Filling, Not Fattening,
    24–31
  Fiber Facts, 28
  Fiber: Good for What Ails You, 26–27
  increasing amount in your diet, 28–29
  list of high-fiber/low-calorie and
    low-fiber/high-calorie foods, 26
  list of nutritious switches, 31
  Outstanding Fiber Foods, 27–28
  Practice: Focus on Fiber, 32
  Practice: Refocus on Fiber, 63
  recommended quantity, 28
  Shopping with Fiber in Mind, 29–31
Fit or Fat by Covert Bailey, 8
Fitness, 39, 42–43, 48, 165
  Fitness Logistics, 54–55
  Fitness Walking Test, 54, 170–173
  Fitness: Beyond Good Intentions, 96–103
  Living Fitness, 53–58
Flinders, C., 174
Flour, white and whole wheat compared, 27
Folacin, 120
Food as Fuel, 56–58
Food Groups, Living Lean Good Food Guide
  Extras, 69–70, 74–75
  Fat, 68–69, 73
  Fruit, 68, 72–73
  Hidden Fat, 69, 73–74
  Milk, 68, 73
  Protein, 67–68, 71–72
  suggested minimum daily portions, 78
  Vegetable, 68, 72
  Whole Grain/Starch, 67, 70–71
For Fleet Athletes, 58
Formula, Living Lean Success. See Success
    Formula

Free To Choose, 119
Fructose, 158
Fruit
    in Good Food Guide, 68, 72–73
    list of high-fiber, 28
    recommended daily servings, 25, 78
    recipe: Festive Fruit Sauce, 155
Fuel-Efficient Carbos, 57

Gallup survey, exercise, viii
Gazpacho, blender (recipe), 36, 140
Get a Line on Labels, 12–15
Getting the Best of Sugar, 158
Glucose metabolism, 157
Glycogen, 8, 57
Good Food Guide
    food groups, 67–75
    how it works, 66
    records, daily and weekly, 78–79
Grain and Bean Cuisine, 31–32
Grains, whole; list of, 27
Gravy, Low-Fat (recipe), 77
Grazing, 33–34

Heart rate, 49, 54
    monitoring during exercise, 49–50
Hearty Black Beans, 31
Herbs, cooking with, instead of salt, 61, 62
Home Cooking (salt, sugar, and fat), 75
How Much Fat is Too Much Fat?, 10
Hunger. See Appetite control
Hunger Busters, 34
Hypertension, 6

Initiative, 1–2, 162, 165
Insulin, 156, 157
Iron, 57, 81, 120, 145
It's About Time, 1–2

Jefferson, Thomas, and walking, 48
Jennings, Dr. Dee, 104
Joel, Billy, 45
Jogging. See under Aerobic activity
Joint stress, 8

Kabobs, cookout, 135
Kidney beans, how to cook, 32
King, Dr. Abby, 48

LABEL LINGO
    fat content, 74
    calories, 76
    portion size, 71
    salt and sugar, 13
    sodium high in some low-fat products, 72
    unbleached wheat flour, 30
    enriched flour or cornmeal, 30
Lactose, 106
Lappe, F., 174
Lean Bean Cookery, 32
Lean Protein List, 72, 114
Lentil-sesame burgers, 129

Lentils, how to cook, 32
Lima beans, how to cook, 32
Living Fitness, 53–58
Living Lean
    alumnus' letter of appreciation, xiv–xv
    participants in, vii–viii
    Participation Agreement, 3
    program summarized, xiii–xv
    Success Formula (Q^2FiT), viii–ix, 44, 83,
        163, 165
Logos, xv
Low-Fat Gravy, 77

Magnesium, 53, 57, 104, 145
Malls, used for exercise, 96–97
Malnutrition, vii
Manganese, 81, 104, 105
Meal frequency and weight gain in growing
    rats, 35
Measurements, body
    personal record, 10
    as life expectancy indicators, 11
Measures, Handy, 71
Measuring portions, 76–77
Medical exam, history, and personal record, 6, 19
Menopause, 104, 105
Menus, ready-made
    1,350 calories/day, 121–126
    1,650 calories/day, 126–132
    2,000 calories/day, 132–138
    2,300 calories/day, 139
    2,700 calories/day, 139–140
Metabolism, xiv, 49, 55, 86–95
    aerobic, 57–58
    decline of, with traditional dieting, 88–89
    effect of spicy foods on, 96
    setpoint, 90, 93–94
Milk
    calcium, amount in, 104
    fat and calories in whole, 73
    in Good Food Guide, 68, 73
    recommended daily servings, 25, 78
    tricks for getting more even if you don't like it,
        105–106
Missing Link, 106, 163–164
Mitochondria, 86
Muffin pizzas, 130
Muffins, Pineapple Oat Bran, 31–32
Muscles, 86

N-Squared Computing, 121
Navy beans, how to cook, 32
Nursing women, calorie-skimping not
    recommended for, 7
Nutrition. See Eating; Good Food Guide
Nutrition Checkup, 25
Nuts and seeds, list of high-fiber, 28

Oat bran, ways to use, 30
Obesity
    a malnutrition problem, vii
    risks of, 7–8

Obstacles to Living Lean program success, 2
Ohio State University, 88
Options for Living Lean eating, 113, 120
Orange Snow, 106
Osteoporosis, 104
Outstanding Fiber Foods, 27–28

Pantothenic acid, 145
Pantry Inventory, xiii, 13–14
Parfait, nectarine-blueberry, 139
Participation Agreement, 3
Parton, Dolly, 45
Pea and Potato Curry, 79–80
Peas, split, how to cook, 32
Personal Time Out, 103
Picante dip, 121
Pinch test for body fat, 10
Pineapple Oat Bran Muffins, 31–32
Pinto beans, how to cook, 32
Plateau profile, 93
Popcorn Parmesan, 36
Portions
    Portion Plans (tables) for women, for men, 115
    Portion Practice, 76–77
    suggested minimum daily, from Good Food
        Guide (table), 78
Positive Person Test, 5–6
Positively Speaking (and Thinking and Doing),
    4–5
Potassium, 57, 62, 72, 145
    amount in certain foods, 60
Potato recipes
    Baked Fries, 36
    Potato crisps, 36
    Potato pancakes, 138
PRACTICE
    Aerobicize Your Schedule, 58–59
    Fill in the Snack Gaps, 37
    Focus on Fiber, 32–33
    Leave One Bite, 140–141
    Moderate Your Meat Intake, 82–83
    Personal Time Out, 103
    Practice Diary, 16–19, 39–41, 63–65, 83–85,
        107–109, 141–143, 159–161, 165–168
    Plan/Record Meals and Snacks, 119–120
    Refocus on Fiber, 63
    Rely on the Good Food Guide, 78–79
    Skimp on Salt, 62
    Slack Off on Sweets, 159
    Slow Down and Savor, 153
    Swing into Action, 101–103
    Taper Off Mr. Caffeine, 39
Pregnant women, calorie-skimping not
    recommended for, 7
Processed vs. unprocessed foods, 60
Progress Evaluation Chart, 12
Protein
    animal, recommended daily servings, 25
    bean-plus-grain favorites, 81
    in Good Food Guide, 67–68, 71–72
    Lean Protein List, 72
    legume, recommended daily servings, 25

Living Lean with Less, 80–83
    needs increased for athlete in training, 57
    personalized protein recommendation, 82
    Protein Pyramid, 81, 117

Q²FiT. See Living Lean, Success Formula
Quality Control Assurance, 66–79
Quantity Control Assurance, 110–112
Quick mixes, high-fiber kinds, 30

Raspberry whip, 132
REA—Recommended energy allowance,
    110–111
Rebound weight gain, 94
    Recipes
    Baked Fries, 36
    Breakfast Sausage, 77
    Cheryl's Sunflower Slaw, 79
    Chris's Kringles, 155
    Eggnog Custard, 106
    Festive Fruit Sauce, 155
    Hearty Black Beans, 31
    Low-Fat Gravy, 77
    Orange Snow, 106
    Pea and Potato Curry, 79–80
    Pineapple Oat Bran Muffins, 31–32
    Spicy Guacamole, 37
    Spinach Dip, 37
    Tortilla Chips, 36
Recipes (simple recipes in menus)
    Apple tea, 36
    Banana French toast, 125
    Banana frost, 140
    Banana-berry smoothie, 125
    Bean-spread pita, 132
    Carob cocoa, 36, 131
    Chef salad, 132
    Chicken, baked "fried" (recipe), 126
    Cinnamon toast, 133
    Cookout kabobs, 135
    Cranapple fizz, 131
    Creole, shrimp or chicken, 132
    Far-East stir fry, 130
    Gazpacho, blender, 36, 140
    Lentil-sesame burgers, 129
    Muffin pizzas, 130
    Parfait, nectarine-blueberry, 139
    Picante dip, 121
    Popcorn Parmesan, 36
    Potato crisps, 36
    Potato pancakes, 138
    Raspberry whip, 132
    Salad, pasta and pine nuts, 138
    Sangrita, 126
    Spanish rice, 137
    Spinach crepes, 128
    Stew, beef or venison, 136
    Strawberry milk, 122
    Stuffed tomato-pepper, 133
    Summer punch, 36
    Tacos, egg and potato, 139

Tapioca, 133
Tofu hamburger, 130
Tomato-buttermilk cocktail, 36
Trail mix, 36
Tuna salad, 128
Turkey taco, 121
Wake-up-smoothie, 133
Yogurt, coffee, 136
Yogurt, maple-nut, 135
Recommendations
    aerobic activity, 55
    calorie intake daily, 111
    fiber, quantity in your diet, 28
    food group servings daily, 25, 78
    personalized protein, 82
Red beans, how to cook, 32
Robertson, L., 174
Rockport Fitness Walking Test, 54, 170–173
Running. *See under* Aerobic activity
Ruppenthal, B., 174

SAD (Seasonal affective disorder), 148
Safety in exercising, 50–53, 96–97
Salad: pasta and pine nuts, 138
Salmon, amount of calcium in, 105
Salt, ix, 13
    Salt of the Earth (list of salty foods), 60–61
    Salty Deceivers, 59
    slacking off suggestions, 61–62
    Shake It Easy, 59–62
Sample Good Food Guide Tallies, 115
Sangrita (recipe), 126
Sausage, Breakfast, 77
Scale weight, 9–10, 91, 163
Set the Timing: Graze, Don't Gorge, 33–34
Setpoint, metabolic, 90, 93–94
Silicon, 104
Sizing Up Meat Portions, 72
Skiing, cross-country, 46
Slaw: Cheryl's Sunflower Slaw, 79
Small Steps Add Up, 101
Smoking, 43–44, 65
Snappy Snacks, 35–36
Sodium. *See* salt
Soft drinks, amount of caffeine in, 38
Some Like It Hot!, 96
Some Sweet Things, 155
Sorensen, Jacki, 45
Spanish rice, 137
Speed Eating Is Not a Sport, 151–153
Spice It Right, 61–62
Spice Up Your Life—Without Salt, 62
Spicy Guacamole, 37
Spinach crepes, 128
Spinach Dip, 37
The Spoilers, ix, 34, 104, 148, 156
    See also Alcohol; Caffeine; Salt; Sugar
Stanford University study, 48
Starch, in Good Food Guide, 67, 70–71
Step Outside, 148
Stew, beef or venison, 136
Strawberry milk, 122

Stress, 144–150
Stretches, 50–52
Stuffed tomato-pepper, 133
Substitution pyramids, 117
Success Formula (Q^2FiT). *See under* Living
    Lean
Success: Don't Settle for Less, 165
Sucrose, 158
Sugar, ix, 13, 56, 153–159
    Choosing a Sweetener, 157–158
    Getting the Best of Sugar, 158
    Practice: Slack Off on Sweets, 159
    Shakedown on Sugar, 156–157
    Stalking Simple Sugars, 153–155
Summer punch, 36
Swear Off the Scale, 9–10
Sweeteners, 157–158
    artificial, drawbacks of, 157
Swimming. *See under* Aerobic activity

Tacos, egg and potato, 139
Tacos, turkey, 121
Tame Your Appetite, 33–35
Tapioca, 133
Tea, amount of caffeine in, 38
Thermogenesis, diet-induced, 95
Thiamin, 57, 81, 156
Time, scheduling, 150–151
Tofu hamburger, 130
Tofu, amount of calcium in, 105
Tomato-buttermilk cocktail, 36
Tortilla Chips, 36
Trail mix (recipe), 36
Training Table Options
    Good Food Guide, 66–83
    Portion Plan, 113–119
    Ready-Made Menus, 120–140
Treasure Map, 3–4, 19
Tuna salad, 128
Turkey taco, 121

USDA study, 26

Vegetables
    calcium in, 105
    in Good Food Guide, 68, 72
    list of high-fiber, 28
    protein in, not as fattening, 80–81
    recommended daily servings, 25, 78
    Very Good Veggies (recipes), 79–80
Vegetarianism, 80–82, 104, 174
Vitamins, 57, 72, 81, 104, 105, 120, 145

Wake-up-smoothie (recipe), 133
Walking, 7, 43, 47–49, 54
    calories burned when, 56
    miles walked in average day, 101
    organized events, 174
    speed, average female, average male, 56
    water required for, 52
    ways to get most out of it, 48–49
    See also Aerobic activity

WalkWays Center, 174
Water loss, 8
Water retention, 60
Week 1, 1–16
Week 2, 20–41
Week 3, 42–65
Week 4, 66–85
Week 5, 86–109
Week 7, 144–161
Week 8, 162–168
Weighing, not recommended, ix, 9–10, 91
West Virginia University, 94
What Do You Want To Lose?, 8–9
What's in a Pound?, 91
What's the Verdict? Eating Diary Analysis, 20–23
What's Your Pleasure?, 145
Whatever Works—For YOU, 162–164
Wheat bran, ways to use, 30
Whole Grain/Starch, in Good Food Guide, 67, 70–71
Wilmore, Jack H., vi, 169
Wine, cooking with, instead of salt, 61
Women, need for positive bone stress, 106–107
Wood, Dr. Peter, 48
Wordsworth, William, and walking, 48
WRITTEN EXERCISES
    Activity Log: A Day in the Life, 100–101
    Are you a Positive Person?, 5–6
    Are You Game for Change?, 2–3
    As the Fat Shrinks, Count Down the Inches, 10
    Assess Your Stress, 145–147
    Be Heart Smart, 49–50
    Breakfast Bottles and Boxes, 15
    Choose to Move, 99–100
    Count on Calcium, 104–105
    Counting Burgers, Beans, and Bananas, 75
    Design a Menu, 117–119

Eating Diary, 16
Eating Habits Checkup, 20–24
Get Up and Go!, 7
How Fit Are You? A Fitness Walking Test, 54
Hurdling Aerobic Obstacles, 98
I Wish I Had Enough Time To . . . , 151
Nutrition Checkup, 25
One Look Back, Full Speed Ahead, 44–45
Pantry Inventory, 13–14
Participation Agreement, 3
Personalized Protein Prescription, 82
Practice: Aerobicize Your Schedule, 58–59
Practice: Personal Time Out, 103
Progress Evaluation, 12
The Progression toward Health and Fitness, xv
Quantity Control Assurance, 110–112
Quick Calorie Check, 114
Salt of the Earth, 60–61
Something Ventured, Something Gained, 164–165
Stalking Simple Sugars, 153–155
Stress RX, 148–149
Take Time to Make Time, 150
Walk It Off, 56
Aerobictips
    Fun with Fitness, 53
    Get Fit on Foot, 48–49
    No Strain, No Pain, 45–46
    Pedal Pushing, 47
    Swim and Trim, 46–47

Yogurt
    amount of calcium in, 104
    coffee (recipe), 136
    maple-nut (recipe), 135

Zinc, 57, 81, 104, 105, 120, 145, 156

ABOUT THE AUTHOR

Cheryl Jennings-Sauer earned a master's degree in nutrition from the University of Texas at Austin in 1980 and is now a registered and licensed dietician. She maintains a private practice, Nutrition-Link Consulting, and serves as Instructor of Human Nutrition at Austin Community College.

Since 1982 her Living Lean seminars and corporate workshops have expanded to include the **Living Lean and Fit**™ program and **Living Lean Cuisine**™ for healthy cooking and dining out. Cheryl also stays busy as a freelance writer for national magazines and as guest host on "The Good Life" call-in health and nutrition radio show.